HOT Flash to HOT DAMN!

The Precision Hormone Program for Perimenopause and Menopause—Reclaim Your Energy, Body, and Self

Amber Bocknek, MD CCFP ABAARM FAAMM MSCP

FREE WORKBOOK

INCLUDED WITH YOUR COPY OF HOT FLASH TO HOT DAMN!

Here's what you'll find inside the **HOT Flash to Hot Damn! Implementation Workbook**:

✓ **Daily Cortisol Reset Toolkit:** Six evidence-based techniques to interrupt your stress response in real time, chosen for the woman whose day never slows down. Includes a one-page personalised plan you can follow without changing your whole life.

✓ **Symptom-Chasing Trap Audit:** Identify which of the three most common traps is keeping you stuck, and get a clear, strategic first step that replaces random experiments with a plan built around your biology.

✓ **Lab Prep & Insight Workbook:** Organise your symptoms in clinical language, track cycle changes without obsessing, and walk into your next appointment with the right questions in the right order.

✓ **Appointment Preparation Worksheet:** Apply the Three-Goal Rule before every visit so you stop leaving with a shrug and start leaving with a next step, a plan, and a follow-up committed before you reach the door.

✓ **Hormone Harmony Follow-Through Plan:** Spot patterns, stay consistent, and build the feedback loop that turns partial improvement into real, lasting change across all four sex hormones.

✓ **4-Layer Reset Checklist:** See all four layers of the midlife reset in one place, identify the single most meaningful first step from wherever you are standing right now, and let everything else compound from there.

✓ **6-Pillar Healthspan Audit:** A self-assessment across all six pillars of elevation that shows you clearly where you are thriving, where there is room to grow, and where your best first step lives.

✓ **Partner Support Guide (Bonus):** A warm, honest, and occasionally funny guide for the significant other of the woman reading this book. Because the people who love her deserve a roadmap too.

Scan the QR code below or visit: www.hotflashtohotdamnbook.com/workbook

GET THE WORKBOOK

SCAN HERE

HOT Flash to HOT DAMN! The Precision Hormone Program for Perimenopause and Menopause — Reclaim Your Energy, Body, and Self

 For permission requests, please contact: Amber Bocknek, MD Suite 105, 15017 Yonge Street Aurora, Ontario, Canada L4G 1M5 DrAmberBocknek@gmail.com

Medical Disclaimer

This book is intended for informational and educational purposes only. It is not a substitute for professional medical advice, diagnosis, or treatment. The content in this book reflects the author's clinical experience, research, and professional opinion and is designed to support — not replace — the relationship between a patient and her healthcare provider. Always consult with a qualified healthcare professional before making changes to your health routine, starting or stopping medications or supplements, beginning any new wellness program, or making decisions about hormone therapy or any other medical treatment. Individual health outcomes vary significantly based on personal medical history, genetics, lifestyle, and other factors unique to each person. **While the author is a licensed physician, reading this book does not create a physician-patient relationship. The information provided applies generally and may not reflect the most current clinical guidelines or be appropriate for your specific circumstances, medical history, or jurisdiction.** The author and publisher are not liable for any adverse health outcomes, negative effects, or consequences — direct or indirect — resulting from the use of or reliance on the information in this book. If you are experiencing a medical emergency, please contact emergency services immediately.

General Disclaimer

The frameworks, strategies, and recommendations in this book represent the author's experience, research, and professional opinion. Results vary based on individual circumstances, effort, medical history, and factors beyond the author's control. The author makes no guarantees regarding specific health outcomes or results. The examples and patient vignettes in this book are composites drawn from clinical experience. Names and identifying details have been changed or are fictional. Any resemblance to specific individuals is coincidental.

Permissions and Attribution References

Permissions and Attribution References to clinical studies, research, and medical guidelines are included for educational purposes. The Women's Health Initiative and other studies referenced in this book are the work of their respective authors and institutions. All such references are used in accordance with fair dealing provisions for educational and informational purposes. The Precision Hormone Program, the Four-Layer Reset, the CLEAR Framework, and other frameworks presented in this book are original works of the author.

Edition Information

Title: HOT Flash to HOT DAMN! The Precision Hormone Program for Perimenopause and Menopause—Reclaim Your Energy, Body, and Self Author: Amber Bocknek, MD CCFP ABAARM FAAMM MSCP **Edition:1 ISBN Audiobook: 978-1-0675638-3-7, Digital: 978-1-0675638-2-0, Paperback:978-1-0675638-1-3 and Hardback Edition:978-1-0675638-0-6 Published: April 2026** ***Printed in Canada*

Well-behaved women seldom make history.

- Laurel Thatcher Ulrich

Foreword

By Dr. Alvin Pettle, F.R.C.S. (Obs/Gyn) (C)

As a male gynecologist who has had the privilege of assisting women through the many years of hormonal havoc, I am delighted to introduce to the world a woman physician — Dr. Amber Bocknek — who has written a new and exciting book that personally elucidates the complex hormonal issues of perimenopause and menopause. She has also brilliantly added a working journal so the reader can follow through these very difficult years with proper guidance. The combination of this unique book and its working journal is pure genius.

Dr. Amber Bocknek states quite accurately that *"our medical system is remarkably poorly equipped to address the management of perimenopause and menopause."* She further writes that *"estrogens, progesterone, testosterone, and cortisol do not decline gracefully on a schedule. They fluctuate, drop, spike, and interact with each other in ways that affect sleep, mood, energy, body temperature, brain function, libido, and a woman's sense of herself."*

I graduated from the University of Toronto Medical School in 1969 (Alpha Omega Alpha) and completed a four-year residency in Obstetrics and Gynecology in Toronto. I was appointed a staff member at Etobicoke General Hospital in the summer of 1974 (now the Sir William Osler Centre). Over the next 20 years, I successfully delivered over 5,000 babies and was the pioneer of the Leboyer technique — the method of water birth — in Canada. It was also at EGH that I met my wife, Carol, the one who truly saved my life. When I first met her, she was the third nurse on the left while I was giving a lecture on Estriol — and I truly could not continue talking when I saw how beautiful she was. For me not to talk is really something.

In 1994, when I was Chief of OBS and GYN at EGH, I took six months off to be with my son Adam, who successfully survived an advanced thyroid cancer with secondaries in his lung. Thanks to Dr. Ian Witterick and the late, great Dr. Paul Walfish, along with the nursing staff at the new Mount Sinai Hospital, Adam pulled through. However, during the radical surgery, they had to cut Adam's recurrent laryngeal nerve, and this left his voice hoarse. He went on to become a successful playwright and wrote, *"I awoke from surgery with a new pair of eyes,"* which is exactly how I felt when I returned to practice after studying bioidentical hormones during those six months off. I became the Canadian pioneer gynecologist who strongly advocated for natural hormones, not synthetics.

In 1995, French scientists discovered how to make natural progesterone digestible. But in 2002, when the WHI study examined synthetic oral Premarin (horse urine) and the synthetic progestin Provera, physicians became confused and largely decided it was safer for them not to prescribe any hormones at all. As Dr. Gilbert once put it: *"There has been an abysmal misunderstanding by doctors of the difference between synthetic progestin and natural progesterone."*

As a practicing gynecologist for 50 years, I have read many books before — but this one, and its accompanying working journal *Hot Flash to Hot Damn!*, impressed me so much that I asked to write the foreword. The author, Dr. Amber Bocknek, has made this her own personal journey — the journey of every woman going through perimenopause and menopause. It is honest, factual, and filled with unique ideas about perimenopause and menopause, written in such a relaxed style that it perfectly matches the personality of this bright, unique, and personable physician and author.

I have always known that women are more intelligent than men, and far more perceptive and intuitive. It has been my honor to help guide and treat the hormonal havoc known as perimenopause and menopause. With this book, Dr. Amber Bocknek has given us an abundance of new material to help guide all of us.

Dr. Amber Bocknek's book begins by placing the hormones we are investigating in order, and in language that can be clearly understood. And with each chapter comes a journal in which the reader can participate in the management of her own health. What a brilliant idea — the writer and the reader meeting each other within the content of the book and journal. Cortisol, thyroid (with the need for more thorough testing), sex hormones, and the body's metabolism — all are necessary to understand when making sense of the multiple symptoms of perimenopause and menopause, especially weight gain, sleep disturbance, hot flashes, anxiety, depression, frustration, and total fatigue of the body. Of course, the author blends this with the multiplicity of roles a woman must play for other people before she takes care of herself — and how difficult it is for a woman to say no to anybody.

I must admit, this man has had to learn that saying no is a necessity of preservation.

I am truly impressed that the author, at her young age, has recognized the need for thorough thyroid testing. I have found over the years that one in four women will have thyroid antibodies and the Hashimoto gene, which explains a great deal of their weight gain.

Through the middle chapters of this unique, original work, the reader begins to feel an elevation of spirit and a kindred connection to the writer, who stays personal and pertinent throughout. As you travel peacefully across the pages, there is a feeling of belonging and a new, intimate self-knowledge that is truly empowering.

The author's knowledge of skincare is unique, and her routines to safeguard your skin are outlined in detail — as practical as brushing one's teeth. You will fully understand what I mean once you read the book and follow her suggestions. You will also see, by keeping score at the beginning of the book and again near the end, the logic and sequence of your advancement — and it will be tremendously liberating.

As we near the end of the book, we begin to realize that when we finish, we are going to miss a very good friend. But wait — Dr. Amber Bocknek remains available to you, and to me, even after we have closed the last chapters. She has wisely made herself available to the reader. We feel the rising of spirit and soul, like the Phoenix once risen from its own ashes. In fact, her closing chapters illustrate this rising up, just as the Phoenix once did.

Reader, I know with certainty that if you use bioidentical hormones, you will awaken your body to move and rise. However, by taking Dr. Amber Bocknek's book home with you today — who knows?

"Shall we dance?"

— Dr. Alvin Pettle

Acknowledgments

There are a lot of people to thank for this book. Partly because it took a long time, and partly because I apparently cannot get through a major life event without accumulating an impressive support crew. You know who you are. I am grateful for every single one of you.

But some of you need to be named. So here we go.

My lovely husband, Jory. There are people in this world who say things like "marriage is easy when you find the right person." Those people have clearly never been married to me.

You were patient when patience was required - and let the record show, that was a recurring theme. You were directive when I needed direction, which I resisted every single time and secretly needed every single time, and you knew both of those things and showed up anyway. Always listening. Always there. Always believing in me on the days I had nothing left to believe in myself with.

Here is what did not make it into any chapter: you see me. Not the performance. Not the credentials or the competence or the "tough cookie" face I have been perfecting since the seventies. The actual underneath - the deep stuff I keep behind seven layers of deflection and a very well-rehearsed laugh. I have worked hard to make that version of myself invisible. You find it every time. You sit with it. You stay.

You married someone who came with complications and plot twists and you never once treated any of it as more than you signed up for. You made it safe to be a work in progress. You made it safe to write this book.

That is not a small thing. That is the whole thing.

Love you forever and always.

The Tim Hortons Drive-Through Lady on Hwy 89 in Cookstown. You handed me my large coffee every single morning with a smile that somehow made the caffeine hit harder. You had no idea you were fueling a physician in the early stages of an autoimmune thyroid storm who had diagnosed herself with too much coffee. Thank you for showing up every day.

The Team at Stevenson Memorial Hospital. The doctors, nurses, and staff who tolerated my clicky walk down the hallways, my increasingly dramatic eyes, and my enthusiastic declarations that I could handle every patient in the building. You were kind, you were professional, and you never once laughed at me to my face. I remain deeply grateful for the distinction.

My Besties. The people who showed up when things got hard and stayed when things got harder. Who sat with me through the divorce, the diagnosis, the uncertainty, and the long stretch of figuring out who I was on the other side of all of it. You were warm and present and exactly what I needed, even when I had no words to ask for it. You already know what you mean to me. I will say it anyway: everything.

And to the women who shaped me:

There are women who arrive at exactly the right moment and do exactly the right thing, sometimes without knowing they are doing it. Some of them saved me. Some of them showed me what I wanted to become. All of them left marks I carry with pride.

Shelagh Wilson. My manager in Brantford during some of my darkest days - the ones where I was swimming in cortisol soup and barely holding it together. Shelagh greeted me at my car every single morning with a gentle smile, a cup of coffee, and a garbage bag. The coffee was for me. The garbage bag was for the state of my vehicle, which had become a rolling monument to a woman in crisis. She never once commented on the chaos. She just quietly cleaned it up and walked me inside. That is a particular kind of love, and I have never forgotten it.

Liesbet Jansen. My colleague, former chief of my department at Stevenson Memorial, and an ongoing friend. Large and in charge, brilliant, deeply caring, and the woman who listened to my stories with patience, ordered the CT scan of my head when I was certain I had a brain tumor, and then gently informed me I did not. She has been part of my sphere ever since, and I am better for it in every measurable way.

Gail Bocknek. My mother-in-law. I want to be very precise about what I am about to say, because Gail will read this, and Gail has opinions.

Gail and I do not always see eye to eye. She advises me - spontaneously, enthusiastically, and from a place of caring, which somehow makes it harder to argue with and I argue with it anyway. She gives me medical advice with the confidence of a woman who has never once let the absence of a medical degree slow her down. She is the quintessential mother-in-law, and if you know, you know.

She is also the mother of the man I love. She is an extraordinarily dedicated grandmother. She was a force in business when being a woman in business required twice the fight, and she is still a force today. For the good and, occasionally, for the more interesting. I do not always agree with her. I always respect her. And somewhere underneath the eye-rolling and the unsolicited advice, I am quietly grateful that my husband was raised by a woman who taught him what a strong one looks like.

Sandi Peterson. My mom by choice. Here is the truth: She was truly a great part of my first marriage, and I claim her for my own. Sandi is a former OR nurse who ran her department the way she runs everything - with authority, competence, and a steadiness that could anchor a ship in a storm. She is a wonderful grandmother, a solid-as-a-rock human being, and proof that family is sometimes something you choose to keep rather than something you are born into.

Marie Lacroix. I am fairly certain Marie is my sister from a different life. She is self-made in the truest sense - everything she has, she earned. Smart, funny, altruistic, and determined in a way that makes you want to work harder just by being in the room with her. I work alongside her now as a consultant, and what I admire most is this: she is exactly the kind of woman I want to be in the work. When someone makes you raise your own bar simply by existing, you should probably thank them. So. Thank you.

Joy Houston. The woman who inspired me to write this book. I crossed paths with Joy only recently, and she is one of those people who makes you wonder how you managed before they arrived. Creative, kind, delightful, and possessed of the kind of quiet determination that moves mountains without making a fuss about it. She saw something in this project before I could fully see it myself, and her belief gave it legs. This book exists in part because Joy Houston showed up in my life at exactly the right time. I do not think that was an accident.

And finally, to you. The woman holding this book right now.

I do not know your name. I do not know which chapter brought you here, or which sentence made you pause, or whether you are reading this in bed at midnight after another night of not sleeping or in a waiting room before an appointment you are dreading. But I know this: you picked up a book about perimenopause and menopause, and you made it all the way to the acknowledgments page. That tells me something about who you are.

Humor and gratitude are coping mechanisms - healthy ones. They have carried me through the hardest seasons of my life, and they are woven into every page of this book on purpose. If even a fraction of what I have learned, survived, and come out the other side of spills over into your own journey, then every late night, every rewrite, and every moment of wondering whether any of this was worth it becomes the easiest yes of my life.

Preface

A Note Before We Begin

She is my sister. My friend. The woman at the gym who trains beside me without either of us ever exchanging names. My neighbor, the cashier at the grocery store, the woman who hands me my coffee through the drive-through window at Tim Hortons on a crisp winter Tuesday morning. She is everywhere, once you know how to look. And once you know what she is carrying, you cannot stop seeing her.

She is tired in a way that sleep does not fix. She has been told her results are normal, that this is just aging, that she should reduce her stress - as though that were a prescription and not an insult. She has googled her symptoms at midnight and closed the tab before anyone could see. She has wondered whether the woman she used to be - the one with energy, with clarity, with a sense of herself that felt solid and real - is simply gone.

She is not gone. She is waiting. And this book is for her.

Why I Wrote This

I am a physician. Trained in the systems that are supposed to help women like her, equipped with the clinical knowledge that should have made me one of the lucky ones. And then I became her.

After five years of tamoxifen following my cancer treatment, I went directly into peri-menopause. I had every symptom, every struggle, all the quiet bewilderment of a woman whose body had become unfamiliar to her. The medical system I had trained in - trusted, built my career within - did not have answers for me. It left me floundering and frustrated, figuring it out for myself. So I did. Not with Dr. Google, but with conferences, direct training in functional medicine, and years of self-exploration that became self-reclamation. I found my own solutions, acted on them, and never looked back. What I wished for in those early years was a handout - something that laid it all out clearly, written by someone who had been through it, not just studied it. I could not find that book. So I wrote it.

What This Book Is

There are other books about menopause and midlife. What I hope makes this one different is the way it sees you.

You are not simply an estrogen-and-progesterone-deficient individual. You are a whole person - with a history, a household, a context, pressures and responsibilities that did not pause for your biology. Real help comes from addressing all of it: the psychosocial layer, the hormonal and metabolic layer, and what I call image congruity - the point at which the outside finally reflects the inside. The point at which you look in the mirror and what you see matches who you actually are.

I sit across from women every day in my practice, watching this transformation unfold. Every few months, a woman comes back changed. Not fixed - revealed. The version of herself she always was, finally with room to breathe. That is why I became a physician. It is why I wrote this book.

What I Want You to Know

Before you read a single chapter, I want you to carry three things.

You are worthy. Not because of what you do or who you care for. Simply because you exist. Your worth has never been tied to your usefulness, no matter how long you have believed otherwise.

The status quo is not your future. The fatigue, the fog, the symptoms dismissed and the years of being told this is just aging - none of it is inevitable. The evidence has moved, the medicine has moved, and there is a path forward that most women have simply never been shown.

It takes work. This is a journey, not a shortcut. But it is a journey with a real destination - a version of your life that is brighter, more energetic, more fully yours - and you deserve to arrive there.

My Wish for You

What I most want to give you, before you turn to Chapter 1, is something no clinical framework can provide.

Hope.

Hope that the woman you used to be is not gone - she has simply been waiting. Hope that your future is unwritten and the best of it is still ahead. Hope that somewhere in these pages you will find your own path to the life that is brighter, closer, and more real than anything that came before it.

I know it is possible because I lived it. And I have watched it happen, again and again, for the women who were brave enough to begin.

You do not have to accept this. Better things are possible. And you are worth every single step it takes to get there.

Now let's begin.

With care and conviction,

Amber Bocknek, MD CCFP ABAARM FAAMM MSCP Aurora, Ontario - 2026

Introduction

Where You Are Is Not Where You Are Staying

You are frustrated. Maybe desperate. Worn down by the gap between who you used to be and who you are right now. Somewhere along the way you stopped feeling like yourself. Underneath all of it, there is still a flicker - a stubborn belief that things could be different. That the woman you were is not lost, just waiting.

That flicker is why you are here. And it is right.

But before I tell you what this book will do for you, I need to tell you who I am. Not my credentials - although those are relevant. Who I actually am. Because the reason you should trust me is not a medical degree. It is the fact that I have been exactly where you are sitting right now.

I Missed It. In Myself.

It is a Canadian winter morning - the kind where the sky is that particular shade of bright, impossible blue that only exists when it is cold enough to make your face hurt. Snowflakes are drifting down in that lazy, unhurried way that makes everything look like the inside of a snow globe. I am in my car, in the drive-through line at Tim Hortons, because I am Canadian and this is simply not negotiable, about to collect the single beverage that had - for reasons I did not yet fully understand - become the only reason my body had agreed to get out of bed that morning.

I was a hospitalist at the time. A physician working in a small rural hospital with thirty beds, no specialists, and a forty-minute commute I used every single day to emotionally prepare myself for the fact that I was, for all practical purposes, every specialist simultaneously. I loved it. I was good at it. I was, by every external measure, absolutely fine.

Except that somewhere around this same time, I started to notice something.

After my morning coffee, I felt - and I want to be precise here, because I am a physician and precision matters to me - absolutely jacked up. My heels would click down the hospital corridor with an urgency that suggested I was either very important or very medicated. My hands had developed a slight, enthusiastic tremor. My heart would flutter in my chest. I was sweating in temperatures that did not warrant sweating. My hair - and I say this with the clinical detachment of someone who has since made peace with it - was departing my head in quantities that could generously be described as impolite.

Yet, every morning I would arrive at the nursing station, throw my arms wide, and cheerfully announce to my colleagues that I could take every patient in the hospital, absorb all new admissions, and tackle any additional tasks they had lying around - and I would do all of it with what my team had lovingly begun to call my "crazy eyes."

We laughed about it constantly. I blamed the coffee. I told myself it was the stress of the divorce I had been navigating - the custody conflicts, the financial uncertainty, the beautiful chaos of a blended family, the relentless background noise of worry that I had become so skilled at managing that I had practically convinced myself it wasn't there.

It was not the coffee.

One morning, standing in the shower, the water hitting my face felt sharp in a way I couldn't explain. I raised my hands to cover my eyes and noticed, with a sensation I can only describe as the floor dropping slightly beneath me, that something was wrong. My right eye was protruding.

My first thought was not thyroid. My first thought - the immediate, fully-formed, medically-credentialed thought of a practicing physician - was brain tumor.

The CT was normal. The bloodwork was not.

Graves disease. Autoimmune hyperthyroidism - with a full complement of antibodies that had, apparently, been building for quite some time while I was busy chalking my symptoms up to caffeine sensitivity and the general vigor of a woman who simply loved her job. I had been walking around with a textbook presentation of hyperthyroidism - the tremor, the palpitations, the heat intolerance, the hair loss, the anxiety, the eye disease - and I, a physician with years of clinical training, had diagnosed myself with: too much Tim Hortons.

I would like to tell you that was the end of my education in what it feels like to be on the wrong side of a clinical encounter.

It was not.

Then Came the Fax

A few years later, at forty-six, I went in for a routine check-up. My family doctor thought she felt something on the left side. She mentioned, with what I can only describe as cheerful medical forthrightness, that I was practically fifty - the standard screening age for mammography. I told her not to be so mean about it. She sent me for an ultrasound and bilateral mammogram anyway.

I complied - against my general preference. Against the internal argument I had constructed about why this was probably nothing. Against, frankly, my better judgment - which was, as it turned out, not actually better at all.

Then I got the phone call.

In the particular composure that shock sometimes lends you when you do not yet have permission to fall apart, I asked my family doctor to please fax me a copy of the report. I watched it come through. I was reading it before the paper had fully cleared the tray.

It was obvious. It was cancer.

Surgery followed. A double mastectomy and reconstruction - which I now refer to, with both humor and genuine affection for the technology that gave me a future, as my aftermarket parts. I say that not to minimize it, but because making peace with hard things while maintaining your sense of humor is one of the most useful skills a person can develop.

What followed was tamoxifen. With it, the most complete hormonal disruption a body can experience - induced menopause, overnight, without warning or preparation. I gained forty-five pounds. I lost hair I had already been losing. I stood in my own mirror and did not recognize the woman standing there.

I had a medical degree. Years of clinical training. A career built on pattern recognition and diagnostic confidence.

I still missed it. In myself. Not because I was careless. Not because I was unintelligent. But because my training had gaps I didn't know existed until I fell through them personally - and those gaps cost me in ways that changed the entire direction of my work.

So I went looking for what I had missed.

I found it in functional medicine, in the emerging science of hormonal sequencing, in the substantial and largely overlooked evidence for bioidentical hormone replacement therapy. I discovered the hormone hierarchy - the understanding that cortisol must be addressed first, thyroid second, and the full complement of sex hormones in proper sequence. I retrained. I rebuilt my clinical framework from the ground up.

Then, piece by piece, I rebuilt myself.

Like the phoenix - and I say that without drama, only because the metaphor is genuinely accurate - I rose from my health ashes. Stronger. Better informed. Considerably happier than the version of me who thought she already had all the answers.

I am not speaking to you from a textbook. I am speaking to you from a drive-through line in a Canadian snowstorm, from a shower where I discovered an eye that had no business being where it was, and from a fax machine where I read words that changed the entire course of my life.

I have made the mistakes. I have found the answers. I want you to have the relief I found - without the scenic route I took to get there.

Why Nothing Has Worked — Yet

You have tried things. The diets, the supplements, the wellness influencers with their morning protocols. Maybe you even made it to your doctor - and left with a prescription for something you didn't ask for and a quiet sense of defeat.

Here is why - not as an accusation, but as an explanation. Most physicians have received between one and four hours of menopause-specific training in their entire career, much of it shaped by a 2002 study whose conclusions have since been revised. The system is overwhelmed and operating on outdated guidance. The women suffering most are the ones who trusted it completely and still fell through the cracks.

The fads failed because they were fragments. The system failed because it was not built for this complexity. Neither failure is yours. Both of them brought you here, and here is where things change.

There is a particular kind of loneliness that comes with feeling unwell in ways you cannot prove. You keep most of it to yourself because you have tried to explain it and watched the response - the well-meaning glaze, the pivot to "we're all tired," the suggestion to sleep more, stress less, drink more water. So you perform. You show up. You deliver at work, at home, in every room you walk into. You hold it together so consistently and so convincingly that most people around you have no idea anything is wrong.

You come home and feel like an impostor in your own body.

Then, there are the doctors. The ones who review your bloodwork and deliver the verdict with a calm that borders on the patronizing.

"Your labs are normal." "This is just part of aging." "Every woman goes through this."

I need you to hear me clearly, because I have been on both sides of that conversation - as the physician delivering those words, and as the patient sitting across from the physician receiving them:

- **Normal is not the same as optimal.**
- **"Every woman goes through this" is not a treatment plan.**
- **You are not crazy.**

The Order That Changes Everything

This book offers the complete picture - in the right order, for the first time.

Before hormones, we address cortisol: the stress hormone that governs everything downstream. Then metabolic health: thyroid function, body composition, the changes that have quietly accumulated. Then the full hormonal picture - not just estrogen and progesterone, but testosterone and DHEA, which are equally important and routinely overlooked. Finally, we restore image congruity: the outside reflecting the inside. Not vanity - wholeness. The point at which you look in the mirror and what you see matches who you actually are.

The sequencing is not accidental. Each layer creates the conditions for the next. This is why partial approaches give partial results - and why addressing everything, in order, changes the trajectory completely.

It is called **The Precision Hormone Program**, built around three outcomes I call your Core Wins: feeling energized, being lighter - physically and emotionally - and looking restored from the inside out. Three areas of work. Nine deliberate steps. Sequenced in the precise order your biology requires right now.

You are going to stop chasing. The social media trends, the elimination diets with no evidence behind them, the supplements you purchased based on a forty-five second video. You are going to stop working harder at strategies that are not failing because of your effort - they are failing because they were never in the right order.

What the Other Side Looks Like

You are going to sleep better again. Not the shallow, fragmented half-sleep you have been making do with - but the real kind, where you wake up and the first sensation is not exhaustion but something quieter. Something that feels, with a small amount of surprise, like readiness.

Your energy is going to return. Not the wired, caffeinated performance you may have been substituting for actual vitality, but a steady, reliable baseline that simply exists - the way it used to, before you started having to manufacture it.

The weight that has been accumulating in ways that defy logic is going to start responding again. Because it was never a discipline problem. It was a sequencing problem. Once the right levers are pulled in the right order, your body will do what it was always designed to do.

You are going to look in the mirror and recognize the person looking back.

On the other side of this book, you do not feel younger. You feel restored. There is a meaningful difference. Younger implies going backward - chasing a version of yourself that exists only in memory. Restored means something more honest and more powerful: returning to yourself. A fuller, more informed, more settled version of the woman you have always been capable of becoming. Not despite this transition. Because of how you move through it.

Before You Begin

Most women who find their way to this work have spent so long prioritizing everyone else that they have stopped placing any real value on themselves. Self-care provokes guilt. Her needs wait at the back of the line while everyone else's move forward. Most of the time she does not even see it until someone holds up a mirror.

What most women discover - often with tears they did not see coming - is that they have been living on the belief that their value comes entirely from what they do for others. That belief ends here. What replaces it is the knowledge that she deserves care not because she has earned it, but because she exists. From that foundation, every physical protocol lands differently.

You are not weak for feeling this way. You are not dramatic. You are not fading. You are not failing at something that everyone else is quietly managing without complaint.

You are a high-performing woman in the middle of a significant biological transition, in a medical system that was not built to see you clearly, doing her absolute best with information that was never designed to actually help her.

Of course this has been hard. The deck has been stacked.

If we had grown up in the same neighborhood, we would be the best of friends. I am completely in your corner. I need you to know - before you turn a single page - that you are not too far gone, it is not too late, and the woman you have been missing is closer than you think.

Now turn the page. Not because you are out of options. Not because you have to. But because some part of you - the part that picked up this book in the first place, the part that has never fully accepted that this is just how things are now - knows that there is more available to you than what you have been offered.

Oh girl. I've got you.

Let's get started.

Contents

Area of Work #1: Biology-First Foundation

Stop blaming yourself. Start understanding your body.

Chapters 1 through 5 build the biological foundation—the science of what is actually happening in your body, the sequence that makes it all make sense, and the knowledge that turns confusion into clarity.

By the end of this section, you will understand cortisol, thyroid, and your four sex hormones better than most women will learn in a lifetime of annual physicals.

Chapter One

When Your Labs Are 'Normal' but You Feel Awful

Why You Deserve the Tailored Suit

A quick note: a few different women will guide you through these chapters. Each one is drawn from real clinical experience—real patterns, real moments, real women who sat across from me and said some version of "I don't know what's wrong, but something is." Susan is our first. Natalie arrives in Chapter 2 and doesn't leave. You'll understand why.

Susan is fifty-eight years old. She has spent three decades building a career in healthcare administration that most people would call exceptional—and that she would describe, with a quiet smile, as the result of showing up and refusing to quit.

She is the person everyone leans on when things get messy. She's the one who stays calm. She's the one who always knows what to say next.

Until she didn't.

The meeting was important. She had prepared the way she prepares for everything: thoroughly, methodically, and with enough notes to run the entire project on her own if she had to. She knew the numbers. She knew the timeline. She had rehearsed her key points in the car that morning, clear and steady.

Then, in the middle of a sentence that should have been easy, her mind went blank. Not a small pause. Not a quick search for a word. A full stop.

The room didn't freeze. Everyone just kept looking at her – waiting. Susan, who has delivered boardroom updates for most of her adult life, stood there with nothing in her hands except the sudden awareness that she had no idea what came next.

She pushed through it. Of course she did. She found a thread, grabbed onto it, and finished the meeting on autopilot. She smiled, nodded, did the thing competent women do when they're falling apart internally, and then excused herself as soon as she could without drawing attention. In the hallway, alone, she stood very still.

The thought that hit her wasn't gentle. What is happening to me? The part no one sees.

For weeks – months, if she's honest – Susan has been noticing small shifts she can't explain. Not dramatic enough to call "sick." Not obvious enough for anyone else to see. But constant enough that she can't ignore them.

It shows up in the mornings first. She wakes up and something feels off. She can't name it, but she knows it the way you know your own house – when a door sticks, when the heat isn't quite right, when something is subtly wrong.

The fatigue isn't the kind that coffee fixes. It isn't "I need a weekend." It's deeper than that. By mid-afternoon, she's choosing what she can handle and what she can't. She starts declining things she used to say yes to without thinking. She's rationing energy like it's a limited resource now.

Her weight has shifted. Not twenty pounds overnight – just enough that her clothes feel different, her body feels unfamiliar, and her confidence takes a hit she doesn't want to talk about. She's eating well. She's still moving her body. Yet, she keeps feeling like her efforts aren't landing the way they used to.

Then there's the brain fog. That's the one that scares her. Not because she thinks she's weak. Not because she can't handle discomfort. Because her mind has always been her advantage.

It's the rereading the same email three times and still not absorbing it. It's walking into a room and forgetting why she went there. It's reaching for a word that used to be automatic and finding...nothing.

Susan can handle hard seasons. She can handle pressure. She can handle a full calendar. What she doesn't know how to handle is the feeling that she can't rely on herself. Underneath all of it is a fear she won't say out loud: I have fought my entire life to be taken seriously. If people find out I'm struggling, everything I've built could fall apart.

She isn't only afraid of feeling "off." She's afraid of being exposed. So she does what high-performing women do. She stays quiet. She keeps going. She pretends it's fine. Until the boardroom makes it impossible. She books the appointment. The appointment that breaks trust.

Her doctor orders the standard panel. Thyroid. Hormones. Blood count. Metabolic markers. The usual boxes. A week later, Susan opens her patient portal. One short note is attached to the results: "Everything looks normal. Follow up if symptoms persist."

Susan stares at the screen for a long time. Because she is not fine. She isn't being dramatic. She isn't imagining it. She isn't confused about what her own body feels like. She's been responsible for big decisions for most of her adult life. She knows when something matters. She knows that "normal" doesn't describe what is happening to her.

But the labs say otherwise.

This is where the spiral starts for so many women: if the paper says you're fine, and you don't feel fine, you begin to wonder if you're the problem. You begin to doubt your own judgment. You begin to blame yourself. That is the moment this chapter is here to interrupt.

Normal isn't the same as optimal

Susan's labs may be within range, but they are still telling a story. You just need to know how to read the language.

Most lab "normal" ranges are built to include about 95% of the population. That is not the same thing as "healthy for you" or "working well for you." It simply means your number isn't extreme enough to trigger an alarm.

This is the line I want you to hold onto: Normal is a population statistic, not necessarily optimal at all.

Let's walk through the kind of pattern I see in women like Susan-women who are told they're fine while their lives are clearly changing.

Thyroid: the signal, not just the label

Susan's TSH-one of the main thyroid markers-comes back at 3.8. Most labs flag anything up to around 4.0 or 4.5 as normal. So she "passes."

But here's what TSH really is: it's a signal from the brain to the thyroid. It's the brain asking the thyroid to do its job. A simple way to think about it is like a thermostat. If the thermostat keeps cranking up the signal, it's usually because the house isn't warm enough. A TSH of 3.8 isn't an emergency. But in a woman with fatigue, brain fog, mood shifts, and weight changes, it can be a clue that her system is working harder than it should to keep up. When you look at it alongside her other thyroid numbers-also "normal," but not strong-you start to see a body compensating.

Working. Pushing. Keeping the lights on.

Menopause transition: the early shift most women are never told about

Now layer in what's happening hormonally. In perimenopause and menopause transition, a common pattern looks like this:

- FSH begins to rise (the brain pushing the ovaries harder)
- Estrogen begins to drop over time (sometimes slowly, sometimes unevenly)
- Progesterone often falls early and hard (sometimes to almost nothing)

Progesterone is one of the first hormones many women lose. When it's low, sleep often changes, anxiety can rise, and the nervous system feels more reactive. Many women describe it as a "wired but tired" feeling. Not because they're weak – because their body is shifting.

FSH is the brain's "work harder" signal. If FSH is rising, it often means the ovaries are having to work much harder to produce less hormone than they used to. That can happen even when a single estrogen number still looks "normal" on paper.

One more important detail: labs are a snapshot. A single blood draw does not tell you what your body has been doing for months-or where you were five years ago.

This is why so many women feel gaslit. They're told, "Your labs are normal," when what's really true is: Your body is changing. The pattern is there. You've just been given a report without an interpreter.

The muumuu and the tailored suit

This is the metaphor I come back to, especially for high-performing women.

Conventional medicine often operates like a muumuu: one-size-fits-most. It covers you. It technically fits. It was designed to work quickly for a wide range of people. In many situations, that approach saves lives.

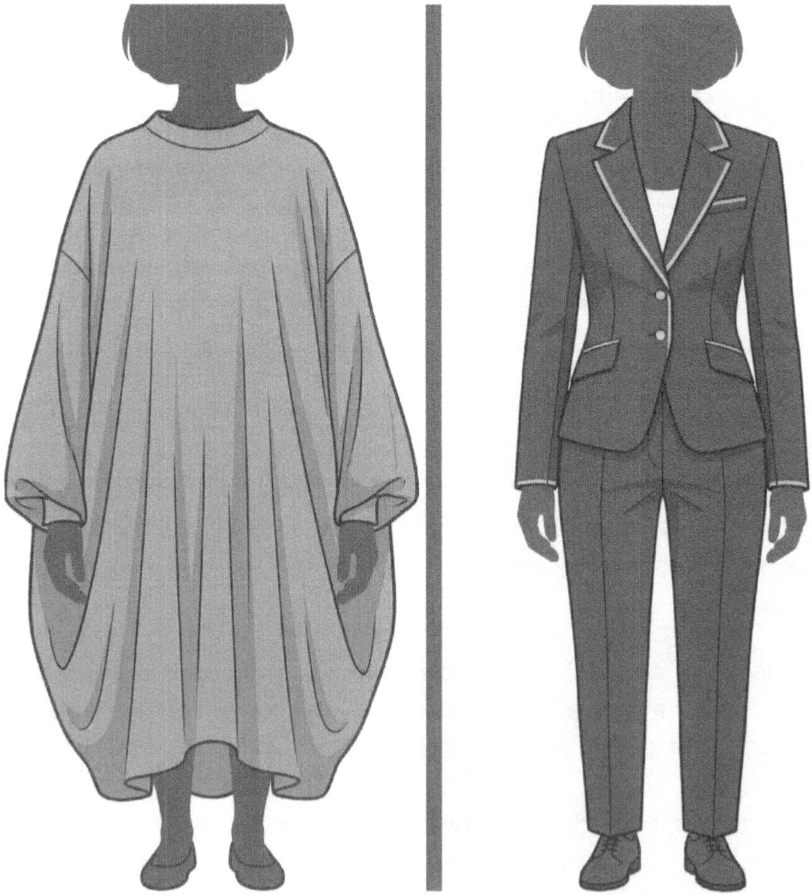

But midlife hormone transition is not a one-size-fits-most situation. It's nuanced. It's personal. It changes over time. It affects the brain, sleep, mood, metabolism, and confidence-often long before anything looks "abnormal" in a basic lab panel.

A precision approach is the tailored suit.

It takes more measurement. More context. More listening. More pattern recognition. But when it fits, you feel the difference immediately – because it was built for you, not the average of everyone.

There's a type of patient who shows up in my office so often I can describe her without ever meeting her. She walks in carrying a binder. Not a folder. A binder. Tabs. Printouts. Highlighting. Notes in the margins. Every lab result she's had for the last several years – most of them stamped normal. Then she pulls out her supplement list. Twelve supplements. Twenty. Sometimes more. Not because she's gullible. Not because she's careless. Because she's trying.

She's been brushed off long enough that she started doing what the system forced her to do: become her own researcher, her own advocate, her own late-night diagnostician. She's full of details – but she's starving for interpretation. She's exhausted. Because effort without clarity turns into anxiety.

The first time a woman like this hears someone say, calmly and clearly, "I believe you," something changes. Her shoulders drop. Her eyes fill. The binder suddenly feels heavier, because she realizes how long she's been carrying it alone.

That's the moment this chapter is designed to give you.

The belief shift

This is the sentence I've said to countless women sitting across from me – women who have been told they're fine while quietly falling apart. The labs are normal. You are not. That line lands because it holds both truths at the same time: Yes, your numbers may be within range. No, you are not okay. That is not a failure. It's information. It's a signal. It's your body asking to be taken seriously.

A permission slip you may need more than you think

You are allowed to stop blaming yourself.

The way you feel is not a character flaw. It is not weakness. It is not you failing at "being healthy." It is biology – measurable, understandable, and addressable.

- You are allowed to trust what your body is telling you, even when a piece of paper says you're fine.
- Your results may be technically normal. But you are not okay-and that is okay.
- You are allowed to ask for more. More answers. More precision. More care that was designed for you.
- You deserve the tailored suit.

The symptom-chasing traps that keep smart women stuck

When a woman is dismissed, she doesn't stop trying. She tries harder. That's where the traps show up – not because she's flawed, but because she's frustrated and unsupported.

Here are three of the most common ones I see:

- The supplement overload. She's taking a lot of things – some helpful, some expensive, some unnecessary, and some that don't mix well together. Most weren't chosen as part of a plan. They were chosen as hope in a bottle.
- Social media diagnosing. She's saving posts. Taking quizzes. Following ten different experts who contradict each other. She's trying to "figure herself out" in a scroll that never ends. The result is rarely clarity. More often it's anxiety.
- Doctor hopping. She keeps switching doctors or clinics – not because she's dramatic, but because she's trying to find someone who will look up from the screen, listen, and connect the dots. When you're dismissed repeatedly, you start looking for a door that opens.

These are understandable responses to a system that keeps saying "normal" while your life says "not normal."

The shift is simple: Stop running random experiments on yourself. Start using a systematic approach built around your specific biology. That is what this book is going to give you.

Why the order matters: hormone hierarchy in plain language

There is a sequence to this work. Hormones don't function as separate little islands. They function as a chain of command. The top of that chain is stress physiology-cortisol. There's a reason for that.

Our ancestors survived because the stress response worked. If a predator showed up, your body needed to mobilize energy immediately. That survival system didn't care about glowing skin, perfect digestion, or libido. It cared about staying alive.

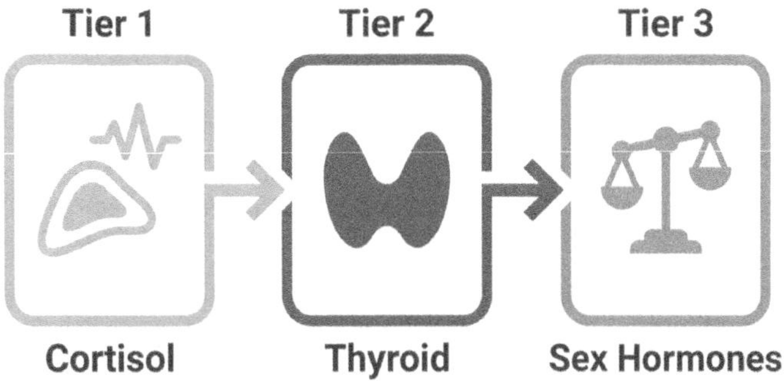

If you were about to be eaten by a sabretooth tiger, it was not a good time to make babies. So when cortisol is high for long periods, it can suppress thyroid function and disrupt sex hormones. It can change sleep. It can change mood. It can change metabolism.

It also affects the immune system over time. Prolonged stress isn't "in your head." It's chemistry. It's a survival state that can wear the body down.

This is why the hierarchy matters: Cortisol first. Thyroid second. Sex hormones third. When you address these out of order, results are often partial and short-lived. When you address them in the right order, the gains build on each other.

We'll go deeper into this later. For now, you only need one takeaway: There is a sequence. It matters.

What Susan leaves with-and what you should leave with too

Susan didn't leave that first appointment with a solution. She left with something more basic, and often more important at the beginning: Validation. A name for what was happening. An explanation for why the things she had tried weren't working. The relief of knowing she wasn't imagining it. She left knowing: What she's feeling is real. It was never "all in her head." It's measurable. It's changeable. There is someone who believes her.

Susan came back three months later. Not with the binder—with one page of notes and a different kind of quiet. She had found a provider who looked up from the screen. The labs were the same numbers. The conversation was completely different. She left with a plan.

If you have felt dismissed, minimized, or quietly ashamed of what you can't "push through" anymore, let this land:

Your instincts have been accurate.

In the next chapter, I'm going to show you how we approach this with structure-so you're not guessing, scrolling, or blaming yourself. You'll get a clear framework for what to focus on first, and why.

The Symptom Clarity Assessment – Your Chapter 1 Resource

If Susan's story feels familiar-if you've been collecting information, buying supplements, switching providers, and still feeling unseen-the first step is not another purchase or another protocol. It's clarity.

The companion workbook turns this chapter into action. Scan the QR code below—or go to www.hotflashtohotdamnbook.com/workbook — to access the **Symptom Clarity Assessment**: a guided tool to help you name what you're experiencing and start building the picture your next provider appointment needs.

Chapter Two

You're Not Imagining It

Here is what's actually going on — and it's not your fault

Natalie is fifty-five. Smart. Successful. The kind of woman people assume has it handled. At 10:47 p.m., she's sitting in bed with her phone six inches from her face, the glow lighting up the part of her that still can't admit she's scared.

She has tabs open-sleep advice, hormone charts, supplement stacks, a podcast episode with a dramatic title, and an article that contradicts it. Her cart is full. Her notes app is fuller. On her nightstand, next to the half-finished tea, was her phone—open to a text thread with her daughter that had gone quiet three weeks ago, right around the time her daughter had started her first real job and stopped needing daily check-ins. Natalie told herself she was glad. She mostly was.

On the other side of the city, her mother was in assisted living now, and the calls from that facility came at unpredictable hours, about unpredictable things, and required a version of Natalie that was calm and capable and completely in charge. She was good at that version. She had been practicing it her whole life.

What she could not figure out was where to put the grief—for her daughter's childhood that was simply over, for her mother's sharpness that was slowly going—or why nobody had warned her that the middle of her life would feel like holding two kinds of loss at exactly the same time.

Her labs are "normal." That phrase has been said to her more than once.

Yet she feels awful. Her sleep is terrible. Her brain is foggy. She's irritable in a way she doesn't recognize. She's doing everything right and nothing is working. The harder she tries, the more it feels like her body is quietly refusing to cooperate. Natalie isn't lazy. She isn't undisciplined. She isn't looking for shortcuts. She's looking for an explanation that fits.

The invisible truth is this: What's happening is real, it makes sense, and it isn't your fault.

The misunderstanding that keeps smart women stuck

The most common belief I see in women like Natalie is a two-part trap:

- "If I just eat cleaner and work out harder, my body will fall back into line."
- "If that doesn't work, then this must be the new normal. I should stop expecting more."

Both beliefs sound reasonable. Both are common. Both can keep women stuck for years. Perimenopause and menopause aren't a moral test. They're a biological transition. When that transition is misunderstood, women keep applying more effort to an old rulebook-until the rulebook fails so completely that they start doubting themselves. Not just their bodies. Their judgment. That loss of self-trust is the real cost.

Why the real problem stays invisible (until it becomes unbearable)

This problem hides in plain sight for three reasons-clinical, cultural, and personal.

Clinical invisibility: the "normal range" problem. Many lab "normal" ranges are designed to catch disease, not early dysfunction. They're built from population averages. That means a meaningful shift for you can still look "fine" on paper. A hormone level can drop substantially compared to your personal baseline and still land inside a wide reference range. On the report: normal. In your life: not normal at all. That disconnect is one reason so many women are told they're fine while they feel awful.

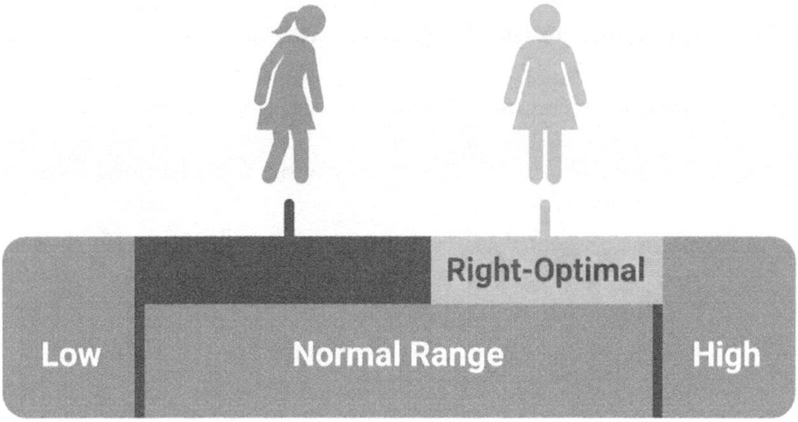

Cultural invisibility: the endurance story. Women are often taught that perimenopause is something to tolerate. A "second puberty." A season to endure. When endurance becomes the expectation, asking for better answers can feel like weakness. Many women go quiet-not because they don't care, but because they don't want to be dismissed. So they carry it privately.

Personal invisibility: the slow drift. This transition is gradual. Symptoms build slowly enough that you adapt. Sleep worsens, so you drink more coffee. Anxiety rises, so you assume it's just stress. Weight shifts, so you cut more food. Focus falters, so you blame your drive. Irritability shows up, so you try to be "better."

You keep adjusting until your body forces a reckoning: insomnia, brain fog, rage, hot flashes, night sweats-something that makes it impossible to pretend this is just a rough month. That isn't weakness. That's your body getting loud enough to be heard.

How I found the invisible truth

Early in my career, I practiced the way I was trained. If the labs were normal, the situation was considered mostly handled-not because I didn't care, but because that's how the system is built: scan the report, rule out danger, move on.

Then I lived the gap between "normal" and "okay." Once you've lived it, you can't unsee it. It changes how you listen. It changes what you look for. It changes how you interpret symptoms-not as noise or drama, but as information.

That experience pushed me to develop a deeper skill set: not just reading lab reports, but noticing patterns over time and connecting them to the woman sitting in front of me-her stress load, her symptoms, her goals, and the reality of her life.

That is the difference between being handed "normal" and being given a plan.

The Precision Hormone Program (high level)

The Precision Hormone Program is for women who are doing everything "right" and still feel like their body is pushing back.

It isn't a pile of tips. It's a structured way to stop guessing and start making decisions that fit your biology and your life.

At a high level, it does three things:

- Better inputs. Not just a basic panel. Not just a generic checklist. We look for patterns that explain your lived experience.
- Better interpretation. Labs are data, not a verdict. You deserve to understand what your results are suggesting-especially when they're technically "normal."
- A clear sequence. So you stop trying to fix everything at once and start addressing the right things in the right order.

The first win: your brain comes back online

The first major win most women notice isn't weight loss or perfect skin. It's mental steadiness. Mental energy becomes more consistent. Focus gets easier. You stop feeling like you're dragging yourself through the day by force. You need less caffeine to function. You crash less often. You can think again.

When that happens, something else returns with it: self-trust. Because brain fog isn't just inconvenient. It's personal. It shakes identity-especially for women whose competence has been their anchor for decades. When clarity stabilizes, she doesn't just feel better. She feels more like herself.

Natalie doesn't need another tab open on her phone. She needs a plan that can turn all that effort into something that finally lands.

Why this approach feels different (and why it's a relief)

Most women have already tried the usual approaches:

- generic "eat less, move more" advice
- symptom-by-symptom fixes
- scattered supplements
- endless research without a plan
- pushing harder because that's what has always worked

The Precision Hormone Program isn't one-size-fits-most care. It doesn't hand you a muumuu and tell you to make it work.

The tailored suit—now with measurements

This is the difference between muumuu care and the tailored suit from Chapter 1—except now we are talking about the measurements. Better inputs. Better interpretation. A plan built for the woman wearing it, not the average of everyone.

What this truth gives you: hope, structure, momentum

Hope. You finally believe relief is possible without more guessing. Structure. You stop second-guessing which symptom to fix first. Momentum. You take action with confidence because you have a clear sequence. When a high-performing woman has clarity and sequence, she does what she does best: she moves.

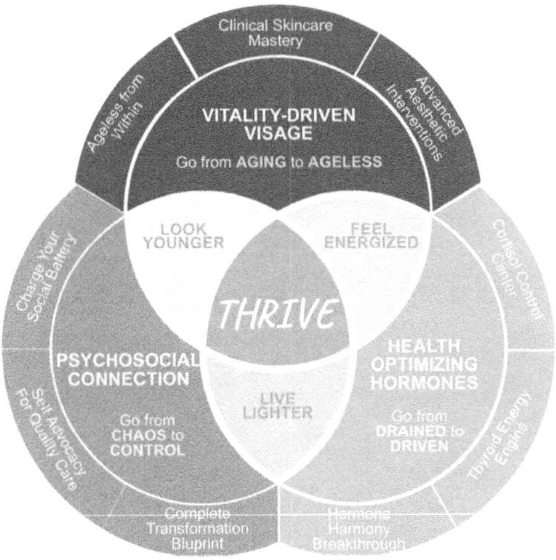

One shift you can make today

When you catch yourself thinking, "I just need to try harder," replace it with this: Labs are inputs. Interpretation is the difference. Strategy is the relief-and it takes more sequence, not more discipline. Self-blame is not a plan. A sequence is.

Your next step – Your Chapter 2 resources

If you've ever left an appointment thinking, "I forgot half of what I wanted to say," you're not alone. When you're tired, overwhelmed, and doubting yourself, it's hard to advocate clearly-even when you're brilliant.

Your Chapter 2 Workbook Resource

The companion workbook turns this chapter into action. Scan the QR code below—or go to www.hotflashtohotdamnbook.com/workbook — to access the **Cortisol Load Reflection Guide:** a practical exercise to help you see your stress patterns clearly and identify where the load is highest.

Chapter Three

Exhausted, But Your Brain Won't Shut Off

Your Daily Cortisol Reset

Andrea is forty-nine. She's a school administrator, married, raising three kids (two teens and one in university), and quietly tracking her father's early memory changes in the background of everything else.

She's the dependable one.

At work, she handles student conflicts, staffing shortages, and emotionally charged meetings with parents. At home, she keeps three lives moving in three directions, makes sure everyone eats, and checks in on her father. She rarely stops. She almost never complains.

But her exhaustion isn't the kind that disappears with rest.

She can go to bed early, sleep seven or eight hours, and still wake up feeling heavy-physically and emotionally. By late afternoon, she's drained in a way that's hard to explain. Small requests feel like too much. Noise irritates her. She snaps more easily, then feels guilty afterward.

Her body starts to show the strain. Weight creeps in around her middle despite unchanged habits. Her joints feel stiff in the mornings-especially hands and hips. Her skin gets reactive during stressful weeks.

Then a pattern appears that she can't talk herself out of: she starts waking between 2 and 4 a.m., her mind alert but useless, as if someone flipped a switch in her brain while the rest of her body stayed exhausted.

What troubles her most isn't the weight or the night waking.

It's the emotional distance creeping into her life. She feels less patient with her children, less connected to her husband, and quietly resentful of demands she used to meet without thinking.

Underneath it all is the thought she doesn't want to admit: Maybe something is wrong with my character.

If you've had that thought, I want to stop it right here. Midlife exhaustion is often not a failure of effort. It's a signal that stress, hormones, and sleep are interacting in ways that require understanding-not more willpower.

That's why the first lever we pull is cortisol.

Stress starts in your mind-but it doesn't stay there

Most women can name their stress. They can list it, schedule it, carry it, hide it, and still perform. But stress isn't only a feeling. It's a body state.

The moment your brain decides something counts as "threat," it sends signals into your body automatically through a system called the autonomic nervous system-your body's automatic wiring. It runs in the background. You don't have to "choose" for it to activate. This is the wiring that influences everyday functions you can't ignore:

- heart rate and blood pressure
- digestion and appetite
- immune signaling and inflammation
- sleep rhythm and sleep depth
- temperature regulation
- mood reactivity and anxiety

This is why "it's just stress" can feel so minimizing. Your body knows it isn't "just" anything. Stress chemistry can affect:

- how easily your heart races
- how shallow your sleep becomes
- how strongly you crave sugar or salt
- how quickly you gain weight around the middle
- how reactive your mood feels
- how inflamed you feel

Your nervous system has two main settings. One part of your autonomic nervous system supports urgency (the sympathetic system). It helps you mobilize, react, perform, and push through. The other system supports repair (the parasympathetic nervous system). It helps you digest, recover, balance hormones, and sleep deeply.

When life keeps you in urgency mode all day, your body struggles to reach repair mode at night-even if you're exhausted. That isn't a mindset issue. It's physiology.

Why cortisol comes first (even when you think your issue is "hormones")

In midlife, many women start by thinking about estrogen and progesterone-and for good reason. Their decline can affect sleep, mood, temperature regulation, and how resilient you feel. But if cortisol is running high, running late, or running unevenly, the rest of your hormone picture can stay stubborn.

Cortisol is your main stress hormone. It exists for a good reason: survival.

The stress system doesn't distinguish between a physical threat and a modern one-an inbox that spikes your heart rate, financial pressure, caregiving strain, or conflict you keep swallowing. The alarm can fire either way. When cortisol stays elevated or out of rhythm, three things tend to happen that matter to almost every midlife woman: Your body stays in survival mode. Survival mode prioritizes vigilance and quick energy. Repair becomes harder to access.

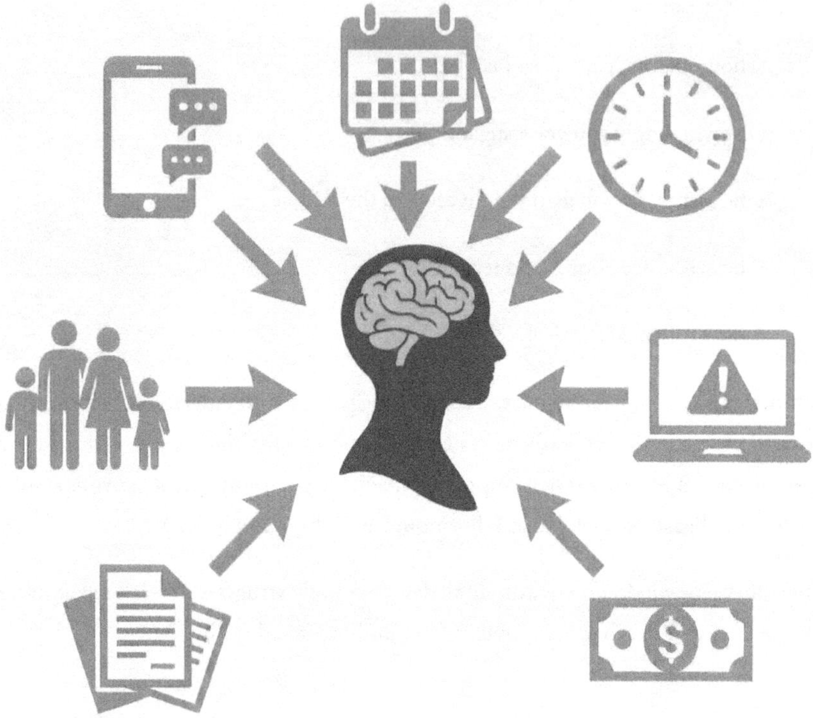

Your sleep becomes fragile. Cortisol and melatonin are meant to trade shifts. Cortisol should be higher in the morning and lower at night. Melatonin rises at night when cortisol falls. If cortisol stays "loud" into the evening, sleep signals don't land the way they should. That's why better sleep often starts with what you do during the day-not only what you do at bedtime.

Other hormones have a harder time gaining traction. Many women get partial improvement when they support estrogen and progesterone, but still feel wired, fragile, or stuck. Cortisol can be the missing piece.

Andrea didn't know any of this at first. She just knew she was trying, and she was still slipping.

Andrea's shift began with relief-not because her life suddenly got easier, but because something finally made sense: Her symptoms were not random. They were patterned.

She learned that chronic emotional load doesn't only live in the mind-it reshapes the body. Years of constant availability can shift stress rhythm, fragment sleep, increase inflammation, and make the hormone transition of midlife feel sharper.

She also learned something high-performing women rarely hear until they're already exhausted: as estrogen and progesterone begin to fall, the stress response can feel louder and recovery can take longer. That doesn't mean you're weak. It means your body is in transition. Instead of trying to push through, Andrea began focusing on regulation:

- treating stress like a biological input, not a character flaw
- protecting sleep depth as foundational
- learning when to slow her nervous system rather than override it

For the first time, rest felt purposeful instead of indulgent. That's the shift this chapter is aiming for. Not "do less." Not "be calmer."

Regulate first. Then build.

The first lever: the Daily Cortisol Reset

You do not need a perfect routine to begin regulating cortisol. You need a reliable way-something you can actually do on a regular day-to help your nervous system downshift.

These techniques work because they change physiology. They aren't about pretending you're not stressed. They're about reducing the stress signal so your body can access repair again.

You don't need all of them. Start with one or two you'll actually use.

A breathing reset (fast, private, repeatable). A simple breathing pattern can shift your body out of high alert. One option is box breathing: inhale, hold, exhale, hold-equal counts. Use it:

- before a meeting
- after a stressful email or call
- when you feel the late-afternoon "frazzled rise"
- when you catch yourself clenching your jaw

Next, A body-based "brake" (when your mind won't cooperate). Your nervous system listens to body cues. A few simple options:

- humming for a minute
- slow belly breathing
- gentle neck stretching
- a brief cold splash on the face

You don't have to do this perfectly. The goal is to teach your body how to downshift.

A transition buffer (so you're not bringing work into bed). Many women go straight from work stress into family demands into bedtime-and then wonder why sleep doesn't arrive. A short buffer between "doing" and "sleeping" matters. Even ten minutes of decompression can help your system shift out of urgency mode.

Sleep support that starts during the day (not only at night). If you're waking between 2 and 4 a.m., don't assume you're failing at sleep. Consider the possibility that your stress system is still active when it should be quiet. Two high-impact moves:

- keep a consistent wake time most days
- create an evening off-ramp (dim lights, fewer inputs, calmer pace)

A modest "digital sunset". Many women are trying to fall asleep while their nervous system is still scanning threats. Start small: turn screens off earlier than you do now. Even 20–30 minutes helps.

Grounding when your brain won't stop spinning. Try this: name five things you see, four you can touch, three you hear, two you smell, one you taste. It brings the brain back to the room you're actually in.

What "done well" looks like

When Andrea began focusing on regulation, she didn't become a different person. She stopped living in a body that felt permanently braced for impact. Her actions were small, but consistent. Instead of overriding the stress state and pushing through, she started interrupting it. She treated sleep depth like a foundation, not a luxury. She learned when to slow her nervous system rather than demand more output from it.

Cortisol-first work looks like this when it's done well:

- you notice activation sooner
- you have a reset you can use in real time
- your evening is less charged because your day wasn't nonstop urgency
- sleep starts to deepen-not perfectly, but noticeably
- mornings stop feeling like recovery from battle

What happens when cortisol work is skipped

When cortisol stays out of rhythm, everything else can feel like it only half-works.

Sleep stays fragile. The 2–4 a.m. wakeups continue. Anxiety stays near the surface. Weight becomes harder to shift. Even when you're doing "all the right things," your body can still feel like it's pushing back-because it's trying to survive, not repair.

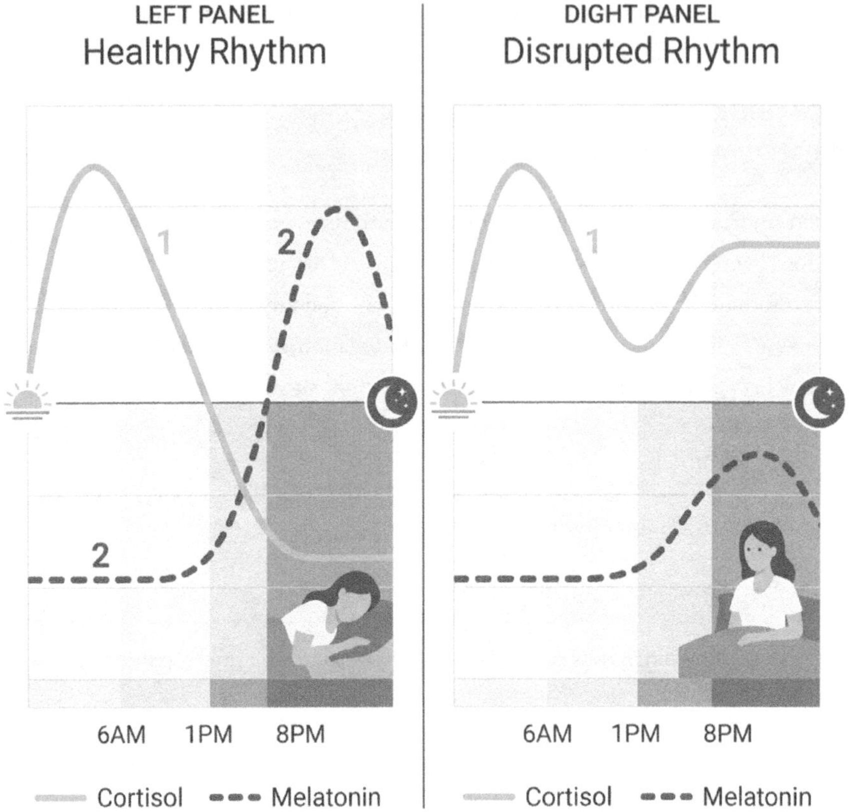

This is also where women become stricter and more self-critical. They tighten control because they're scared. But that often increases the stress chemistry that's already driving the problem.

Cortisol-first work breaks that loop.

Andrea's outcome (and what it teaches)

As Andrea stabilized her stress physiology, her body responded. Sleep deepened. Night waking decreased. Morning stiffness eased. Her mood steadied. Her skin became less reactive. She felt more emotionally present with her family and less depleted by connection.

What surprised her most was capacity. She didn't become less responsible-she became more resourced. She could show up without resentment because she wasn't running on empty.

Midlife exhaustion is often not a failure of effort. It's a signal that stress, hormones, and sleep are interacting in ways that require understanding-not willpower.

Because it's a system, it can be influenced.

Six weeks in, Andrea stopped waking at 3am every night. Not never—but the nights outnumbered the waking for the first time in two years. She told me the most surprising part wasn't the sleep. It was that she stopped feeling like something was wrong with her character.

If your body has been living in high alert for months-or years-more discipline won't solve it. A calmer baseline will. Scan the workbook QR code to access the **Daily Cortisol Reset Guide** in our workbook. I'll lay out the techniques from this chapter step-by-step, help you choose the ones that match your pattern, and give you a one-page plan you can follow without changing your whole life.

Your Chapter 3 Workbook Resource

The companion workbook turns this chapter into action. Scan the QR code below—or go to www.hotflashtohotdamnbook.com/workbook — to access the **Daily Cortisol Reset Guide**: a practical exercise to help you see your stress patterns clearly and identify where the load is highest.

Chapter Four

The Gear Nobody Checked

Why your thyroid may be the missing piece

Michelle is the kind of woman doctors describe as "doing all the right things." She eats well. She exercises. She keeps the calendar running. She shows up for everyone. Still, her body starts to feel harder to live inside.

Her energy drops. Her thinking feels slower. Weight creeps up even though nothing has changed. Sleep stops feeling restorative. Small tasks take more effort than they should. So she finally says it out loud in an appointment.

The doctor checks one number and replies, "Your TSH is normal."

Michelle nods, because she doesn't want to be difficult. Because she's tired. Because she assumes that if the test is normal, her experience must not be. This is where women get stuck in the grind: the body is sending clear signals, but the evaluation stops too soon.

This chapter is where we widen the lens. Not so you can become your own endocrinologist. So you can understand what your thyroid does, what can go wrong, and why "normal" sometimes isn't the same as "well."

The thyroid's real job: set the speed of your whole system

Your thyroid is a small gland in your neck. But it has a big job. Think of thyroid hormone as your body's metabolic speed setting. A helpful analogy is a thermostat:

- When the thermostat is set too low, the whole building feels cold and sluggish.
- When it's set too high, the building feels hot and uncomfortable.

Your thyroid does something similar for your body. It influences how fast you burn fuel, how warm you run, how steady your digestion is, how sharp your brain feels, and how "responsive" your body feels to the healthy things you're doing.

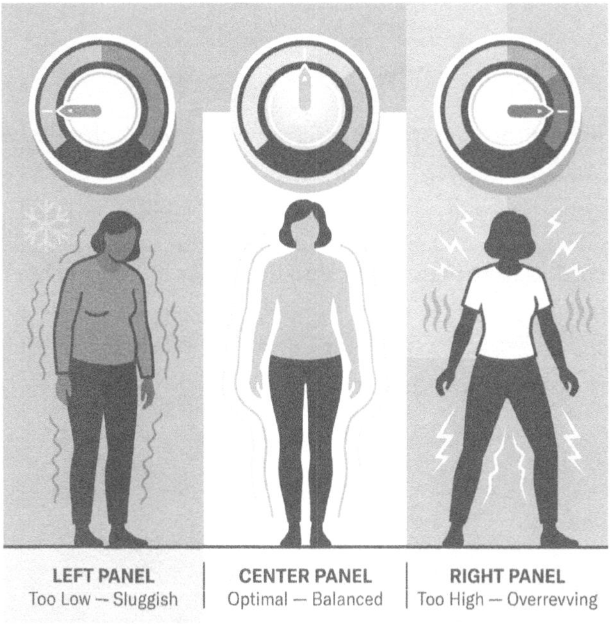

When the thyroid is off, the same woman can eat clean, work out, and still feel like she's dragging herself through her day. That's not a character flaw. That's physiology.

When thyroid is low: the body runs in slow motion – Hypothyroidism

When the thyroid isn't producing enough hormone, the system slows down. Common signs include:

- fatigue that doesn't match your effort
- weight gain or stubborn weight
- constipation
- feeling cold more easily
- dry skin
- low mood
- forgetfulness or "brain fog"

This can feel like you lost your spark. But very often, it's simply that the body is trying to function on a slower setting.

When thyroid is high: the body runs too hot – Hyperthyroidism

When the thyroid is overactive, it can speed up metabolism so much that it stops feeling like "energy" and starts feeling like agitation.

Common signs include:

- heat intolerance (you run hot)
- sweating that feels out of proportion
- heart racing or palpitations
- tremor or shakiness
- trouble sleeping
- irritability, anxiety, or a sense of being "revved up"

Here's what makes this tricky: at first, it can look like stress. It can look like a busy season. It can even look like productivity-until it becomes impossible to ignore. I know, because I lived it.

The part I wish I had understood sooner (even as a physician)

There was a season when I was working in the hospital while my body was clearly over-revving. I had palpitations. I was sweating. My sleep was breaking. My hair was thinning. I felt wired and depleted at the same time.

I did what high-functioning women do best: I minimized it. I also did what physicians are oddly talented at: I went into denial. I didn't want a diagnosis. I wanted to keep being the person who handles things. Then my body escalated. I developed thyroid eye disease-my eye position started to change. It scared me. It was visible. It made "maybe it's nothing" impossible.

That's when deeper testing finally showed the truth: antibodies were involved, and my active thyroid hormone levels were dangerously high. The lesson is simple: A woman can look fine and still be in trouble. One "normal" screening test can delay clarity.

Antibodies: when the immune system gets the wrong target

One reason thyroid problems get missed-or misunderstood-is that sometimes the issue isn't only "how much hormone." Sometimes the issue is the immune system. Your immune system is supposed to protect you. Antibodies are part of that defense. But in autoimmune thyroid disease, the immune system can make antibodies that react to your own thyroid tissue.

In Graves' disease as an example, certain antibodies don't just "attack." They stimulate the thyroid to work overtime. That can drive hyperthyroid symptoms.

A plain-English way to think about it: Your immune system is like a security team. Autoimmune disease is when the security team starts responding to the wrong person. Not because you did something wrong. Because the body is misreading a signal.

Why thyroid eye disease can happen (Thyroid Eye Disease)

This matters because antibodies don't always stay "contained" to one symptom. Some people with autoimmune thyroid disease develop thyroid eye disease, which involves inflammation and swelling in the tissues around the eyes.

Symptoms can include:

- gritty, dry, irritated eyes
- puffiness or redness
- pain behind the eyes
- bulging of the eyes
- double vision
- trouble fully closing the eyelids in more severe cases

Here's the simplest analogy for what's happening: Sometimes the immune system reacts to a "look-alike." The tissues behind the eyeball can resemble the thyroid target closely enough that the immune response spills over.

Doctors have a name for that kind of look-alike mistake: molecular mimicry. You can think of it as mistaken identity.

Most cases improve over time. Some are more serious. In severe cases, people may need special prism glasses or even surgery to relieve pressure in the eye socket.

I'm not telling you this to alarm you. I'm telling you because women are trained to downplay symptoms-and thyroid symptoms are not something to brush off for months while you keep grinding.

The core problem for high-performing women: "screening" gets mistaken for "evaluation"

In many clinics, thyroid testing starts with a screening lab called TSH. TSH can be useful. But it is not always the full story-especially when symptoms persist.

What I want you to take from this chapter is not a list of labs to memorize. It's a principle: When your day-to-day life doesn't match reassurance, you're allowed to ask for a fuller picture.

That brings us to the mindset shift that changes everything: I'm not being difficult. I'm being precise. Precision is not confrontation. Precision is self-respect.

What "early traction" can look like (first 2–4 weeks)

Thyroid progress is often a process, not a moment. If treatment changes are needed, it can take time to fully stabilize. But many women feel meaningful early traction in the first few weeks because the guessing stops and a clear plan begins. Here are three early wins to look for:

- Relief + calm. "This makes sense now." Self-blame loosens because there's finally an explanation.
- Sleep starts to stabilize. Nights feel less wired. Sleep feels less fragile. You may still wake up-but it's easier to settle back down.
- Mood steadies. Less hair-trigger irritability. More capacity inside the same life.

These aren't finish-line wins. They're traction wins-the beginning of climbing out of the grind.

Michelle came back to her next appointment with the **Thyroid Conversation Prep Sheet** printed out and her three symptoms written at the top in pen. Her doctor ordered the fuller panel. The results told a different story than the TSH alone had. She called it the first time in years she had left a medical appointment feeling like someone had actually looked.

Your Chapter 4 Workbook Resource

The companion workbook turns this chapter into action. Scan the QR code below—or go to www.hotflashtohotdamnbook.com/workbook — to access the **Thyroid Conversation Prep Sheet:** the questions worth bringing to your provider and the lab markers worth asking about.

Chapter Five

Stop Telling Me It's Normal

An honest conversation about hormones, desire, and intimacy

Natalie didn't look like someone falling apart. She was the woman who handled things. She exercised. She worked. She showed up. She did the "good girl" version of health: protein, steps, water, supplements, discipline.

And yet, her body was changing anyway.

Weight crept up even though her habits hadn't. Her joints ached in the morning. Anxiety showed up like an uninvited coworker in every meeting. Brain fog made her second-guess herself mid-sentence. So she did what high performers do when something isn't working: she tried harder-and she researched harder.

She added supplements. Switched supplements. Bought better supplements. Listened to more podcasts. Ran more labs. Found more opinions. Instead of feeling more in control, she felt more overwhelmed-like she was drowning in information with no order.

That's the moment this chapter is for.

Because for so many women in perimenopause and menopause, the problem isn't effort. The problem is fragmentation: treating symptoms as separate fires instead of seeing the one system that keeps relighting them. The system that most often gets treated like four separate problems-when it's actually one connected network-is your sex hormones.

The core promise of this chapter (without the hype)

This isn't a "quick fix" chapter.

It's the chapter that helps you stop feeling like you're cycling through versions of yourself-one week wired, one week flat, one week emotional, one week foggy-without knowing why. Precision Hormone Program breaks the start-stop cycle because it addresses the root hormone patterns driving perimenopause/menopause symptoms, instead of asking you to patch over them with band-aid solutions.

Here's the most important thing I want you to hear early: You don't become someone new. You come back to yourself. (Not overnight. Not perfectly. But in a way that's steady enough to trust.)

Why supplement hopping happens (and why it's not your fault)

When hormones shift, your symptoms don't arrive politely in one category.

They pile up: Sleep gets fragile. Mood gets reactive. Your brain feels slower. Your body stops responding to the "right" habits. Your libido disappears. Your workouts feel heavier. Your skin changes. Your confidence takes hits in places no one can see.

So you do what makes sense: you try to solve each symptom as its own problem.

- You try magnesium for sleep.
- Ashwagandha for stress.
- Something for hot flashes.
- Something for energy.
- Something for weight.
- Something for mood.

Sometimes you get a little relief. Sometimes you get side effects. Sometimes nothing happens. Then you assume you chose the wrong thing-or you didn't do it "consistently enough"- so you switch again. That's the start-stop cycle: hope → effort → mixed results → self-doubt → restart.

The Precision Hormone Program doesn't shame that cycle. It simply replaces it with a better strategy: A coordinated plan for the whole hormone network-plus testing and follow-up so you're not guessing.

The big truth most women aren't told: you don't have "one hormone problem"

You have four key sex hormones that act like a team:

- Estrogen
- Progesterone
- Testosterone
- DHEA

Men and women share the same hormones; we mainly differ in levels and ratios. These hormones don't just "live" in the ovaries. Your hormone receptors are spread throughout your body – brain, bone, muscle, skin, and genitals – so when hormones shift, your whole body feels it.

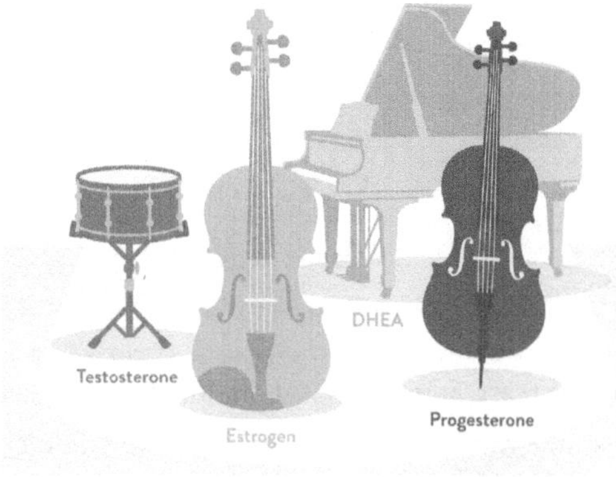

A simple analogy: the orchestra (and why one instrument can't carry the whole song). If estrogen is the lead violin, progesterone is the steady rhythm section, testosterone is the percussion that gives drive and power, and DHEA is the behind-the-scenes support that keeps the whole system resilient-then trying to "fix menopause" with only one hormone is like asking one instrument to play the entire symphony.

It's not that the instrument is bad. It's that the system is incomplete.

What each hormone does-in plain English

This section is intentionally simple. You do not need to become a hormone expert. You just need to understand the job description of each hormone so your symptoms stop feeling random.

Estrogen: the "connection" hormone

Estrogen supports your brain, bones, skin, and temperature control. It influences how "smoothly" your body runs day to day-especially during perimenopause and menopause. When estrogen drops or fluctuates, many women notice hot flashes, night sweats, vaginal dryness, skin changes, and brain fog.

What estrogen shifts can feel like: You're fine...until suddenly you're not. You wake up overheated. You can't regulate temperature. Your brain feels like it has pop-up ads.

Progesterone: the "calm and sleep" hormone

Progesterone supports sleep, mood, and stress resilience. Many women describe the right progesterone support as their nervous system finally getting permission to exhale. In practice, bedtime oral micronized progesterone is often used specifically because it can support deeper sleep.

What low progesterone can feel like: "Tired but wired." Light sleep. Early waking. Anxiety that feels bigger than your actual life.

Testosterone: the "drive and strength" hormone

Testosterone isn't just about libido. In women, it supports bone and muscle, mental drive, confidence, and stamina. When testosterone is too low, women often describe a loss of "edge"-not aggression, but capacity.

What low testosterone can feel like: Everything takes more effort. Motivation disappears. Work feels heavier. You don't feel like initiating anything-conversation, exercise, sex, plans.

The conversation nobody starts: intimacy and desire

I want to pause here, because there is something that testosterone affects profoundly, that most health books treat as either a punchline or a footnote, and that the women sitting across from me almost never bring up first.

Libido.

When testosterone declines—alongside the shifts in estrogen, progesterone, and DHEA—desire often changes. Not always dramatically. Sometimes it just dims. The interest that used to arrive on its own stops showing up. Initiation—of sex, of closeness, of physical contact—starts to feel like effort rather than instinct. The woman who used to want her partner, who used to feel desire as a natural part of her day, quietly wonders what happened to that version of herself.

Here is what I want you to understand: this is not a relationship verdict. It is not a personal failing. It is not evidence that something is wrong with your marriage or your attraction or your identity. It is a physiological shift involving every hormone on this page, plus factors—sleep quality, stress load, body image, vaginal comfort, emotional safety—that no single blood test captures.

It is remarkably common. The majority of women in perimenopause and menopause experience some change in desire, arousal, or sexual comfort. Most do not talk about it—not with their partners, not with their friends, and certainly not with their doctors. They carry it privately, often with shame, often wondering if they are the only one.

You are not the only one.

What is also true: this is addressable. Hormone support—particularly testosterone, but often in coordination with the full picture—can make a meaningful difference. So can addressing vaginal dryness and comfort, which is a separate but related conversation your provider should be willing to have with you. So can sleep. So can the boundaries and energy work coming in Chapter 6, which directly affect whether you arrive at the end of the day with anything left for intimacy—or whether your partner gets whatever crumbs remain after everyone else has been fed.

I am not going to prescribe a solution here, because your solution depends on your specific biology, your relationship, your comfort, and your goals. What I am going to do is name it—clearly, clinically, and without flinching—so that you have permission to bring it into the room. With your provider. With your partner. With yourself.

If there is a conversation about intimacy you have been avoiding, this is your invitation to stop avoiding it. Not today, if you are not ready. But soon. Because desire is not a luxury. Connection is not optional. You deserve to feel like a whole woman—not the version of yourself that runs on logistics and obligation and has quietly stopped expecting pleasure.

That part of you is not gone. She is waiting—and she is part of this work too.

DHEA: the "reserve tank" hormone

DHEA is a building-block hormone that supports resilience-especially under stress. It also relates to immune and cortisol balance. When DHEA is low, women often feel like they have no buffer: normal life feels like too much life.

What low DHEA can feel like: Burnout that doesn't lift. Poor stress tolerance. Feeling "older" faster than your calendar age.

How the four hormones connect (why your symptoms cluster)

Now let's tie it together-because this is where women finally stop feeling crazy. The "night → morning → day" chain reaction

When progesterone is low, sleep becomes lighter. When sleep is lighter, your stress system gets louder. When your stress system is louder, your body is more reactive-emotionally and physically. When your body is more reactive, you become less tolerant to estrogen swings. When estrogen swings hit harder, hot flashes and night sweats disrupt sleep even more.

That's not a character flaw. That's a loop.

The "confidence and capacity" layer. When testosterone is supported appropriately, many women don't just notice libido changes-they notice they feel more steady, more able to handle work and life without snapping. That matters because perimenopause doesn't only change bodies; it changes identity. The goal isn't to "power through." The goal is to rebuild baseline capacity.

The "resilience" layer. When DHEA is depleted, the whole system is less resilient. Your tolerance for noise, conflict, over-scheduling, and poor sleep shrinks. It's like your internal shock absorbers wore out. Again: not moral. Not laziness.

Biology.

The story pattern: why women like Natalie get stuck

Natalie wasn't lacking information. She had too much information-with no sequencing. She did what so many women do:

- She treated the symptoms as separate problems.
- She tried to out-research the chaos.
- She kept changing the plan before any plan had time to work.

Here's what changed her trajectory: She learned that menopause requires order, not intensity. That sleep disruption and inflammation often need to stabilize first. That metabolic shifts are physiological, not moral. Once she had a roadmap, her anxiety eased-not because everything was magically solved, but because she wasn't guessing anymore.

The mistake I see in real clinics (and the moment it finally clicks)

Here's a personal moment from my practice that I think about often: I had a patient who cycled through three different hormone protocols in four months because no one was testing her levels. Every change was based on feelings alone, which meant every rough week looked like "this isn't working." Once we implemented structured, regular metabolite testing and follow-up, she stayed consistent for two years-and finally felt like herself again.

That's the whole point of the Precision Hormone Program: Not endless tweaking. Not endless hoping. A plan, plus feedback, plus enough consistency for your system to settle.

"Test, don't guess": the simplest way to explain hormone levels

Let's make this practical without making it complicated.

The bathtub analogy:

Imagine your hormone level like water in a bathtub:

- The tap is the dose (what you're taking or producing).
- The drain is how your body clears and processes hormones.
- Two women can be on the same dose and feel completely different, because their "drains" are different. One clears quickly. One clears slowly. One makes certain breakdown products that cause symptoms even when blood levels look "fine."

That's why some women say: "I tried hormones and I felt worse," or "It worked for two weeks and then it didn't."

Sometimes the missing piece isn't more hormone. Sometimes it's understanding the tap and the drain.

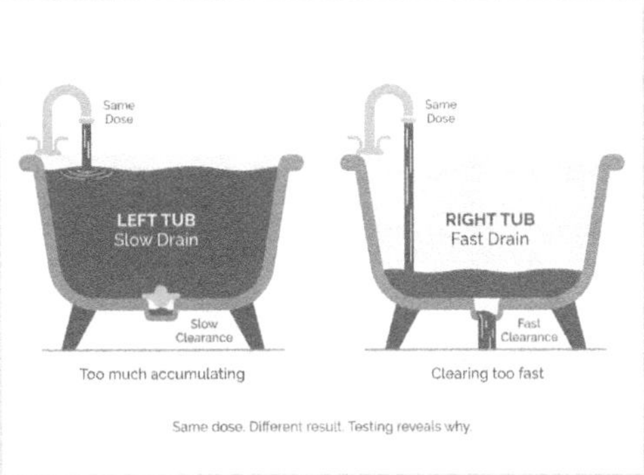

Blood levels vs. metabolite testing (simple explanation)

Traditional bloodwork can tell you what your circulating hormone levels look like right now. Metabolite testing (often urine-based) can show how your body is breaking down and clearing used hormones-your "drain pattern." This can help explain symptoms that don't match what you'd expect from blood levels alone.

This is not a DIY project. Monitoring should be coordinated with a qualified care provider, and many patients do best with scheduled check-ins and periodic re-testing rather than constant changes.

A short, clarifying note on hormone therapy options (because the internet is loud)

There are two practical ideas you need here-not a debate, not a deep dive.

Route matters

First, major menopause guidance notes that transdermal routes and lower doses may reduce certain risks (like blood clots and stroke) compared with oral estrogen in some women. ACOG also discusses that oral estrogen can have a higher clot risk compared with transdermal estrogen.

Second, Progesterone and progestins are not the same thing. Micronized progesterone (often called "natural" progesterone) is not identical to synthetic progestins, and research has discussed different risk profiles between them.

The takeaway <u>is not</u> "everyone should do hormones." The takeaway is: If you're considering hormones, details matter-type, dose, route, history, goals, and follow-up.

If what you heard years ago made you cautious

There is a conversation we need to have before we go further—because I know it is sitting in the room with us, even if neither of us has named it yet.

Many women carry a fear about hormone therapy that was seeded by headlines in the early 2000s. The Women's Health Initiative study made international news, and the message that landed—hormones cause cancer, hormones cause heart attacks, hormones are dangerous—landed hard and stayed.

If that fear has been part of your story, you are not wrong to have been cautious. You were responding to the information that was available to you, and that information was genuinely alarming.

Here is what has changed since then: the clinical conversation has evolved significantly. The original study looked at specific formulations, in a specific population, at a specific time in the menopausal transition. Over two decades of follow-up data and additional research have added considerable nuance—around timing, around type, around route, around who benefits most and who needs a different approach.

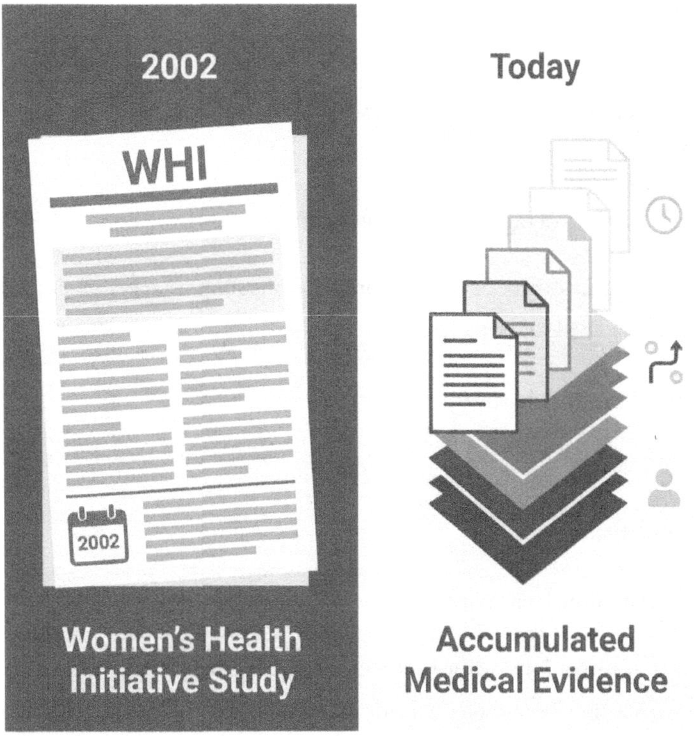

I want you to carry two things:

First, caution and curiosity can coexist. You do not have to abandon your caution to keep reading. You just have to be willing to let the conversation update itself.

Second, the decision always belongs to you. No clinician, no book, and no headline gets to make it for you. What you deserve is an informed, individualized conversation with a qualified provider who is current on the evidence—not a decision made in 2002 based on a news segment you half-remember while brushing your teeth.

That conversation is coming. For now, keep reading.

What "success" looks like (and how to keep it honest)

I'm going to be careful here, because overpromising is one of the fastest ways to lose trust. But it's also true that when women finally get a coordinated plan, the change can be dramatic-not because they became different people, but because their physiology stopped fighting them.

Early stabilization signs (often within 2–4 weeks, for many women).Many women notice two changes first:

- Hot flashes and night sweats begin to drop.
- Sleep improves-especially when progesterone support at bedtime is appropriately matched to the patient.

When sleep improves, a cascade often follows:

- More energy
- Better focus
- Less emotional reactivity

The deeper transformation: By the time some women arrive for help, they don't just feel tired-they feel like they're coming unglued. Anxiety and irritability compound with brain fog until even the highest performer feels derailed at work and disconnected at home. Everything feels like too much, and everyone feels intolerable.

Then-when the system stabilizes-calmness settles back in. Focus returns. Sleep feels restorative. Energy becomes steadier. Irritability softens. Relationships become possible again: with kids, spouses, friends, colleagues.

That's not perfection. That's recognition: "Oh. There I am."

The traps that pull women back into the start-stop cycle

If the Precision Hormone Protocol is the "order," these are the four ways women get pulled back into chaos:

One-hormone thinking. Treating estrogen, progesterone, testosterone, and DHEA like separate problems often creates partial relief and lingering symptoms-because receptors across the body need coordinated support.

"More must be better". High levels can sometimes create symptoms that look like low levels. That's why we don't guess based on symptoms alone. We test, adjust, and re-check rather than chase sensations.

Changing too many variables at once. If you change five things in one week, you can't tell what helped, what hurt, and what was coincidence. Consistency is not boring here-it's how you get your data.

Quitting at 20% improvement. That first "I can sleep again" win is real. But it's not the finish line. The goal is to stay with a plan long enough for your system to stabilize.

Why this step works better after cortisol and thyroid are supported

The Precision Hormone Protocol is powerful on its own-but it works better when the foundation is stable. When cortisol is regulated, your body exits constant alarm mode. Hormone signals can "land" more consistently because receptors aren't being drowned out by stress chemistry.

When thyroid is optimized, your metabolic "engine speed" is steadier-supporting sleep, recovery, energy, and responsiveness. A supported metabolism gives sex hormones more room to work.

The Precision Hormone Program becomes the layer that coordinates the whole body-so you stop feeling like you're managing five emergencies at once.

How to move forward

You have multiple good pathways. The goal is simply this: Get your hormones evaluated as a connected system, with qualified guidance and follow-up-so you can stop guessing.

Here are three clean options, depending on your situation:

- Path 1: Start with your primary care clinician. Bring your symptoms, your history, and ask for an evaluation and follow-up plan. Shared decision-making and periodic re-evaluation are key.
- Path 2: Work with a clinician comfortable with both traditional and deeper testing. Some practitioners use standard bloodwork plus functional testing to better understand the "tap and drain" pattern-dose and clearance-so care is personalized instead of generic.
- Path 3: If you don't have support yet, use the workbook as your bridge. The workbook helps you spot patterns, prepare for doctor visits, and stay consistent long enough to get real feedback instead of false starts.

Your Chapter 5 Workbook Resource

The companion workbook turns this chapter into action. Scan the QR code below—or go to www.hotflashtohotdamnbook.com/workbook — to access the **Intimacy and Vitality Reflection Tool:** a private, honest assessment of where this dimension of your health currently stands and what you want it to look like.

Area of Work #2: Care Focused Connection

Protect your energy. Advocate for yourself. Work with your biology.

Your biology is stabilizing. Now the bottleneck shifts—to the people, obligations, and emotional load that drain you even when your hormones are improving. These chapters give you the tools to protect your energy, navigate the medical system, and build a plan that works with your biology instead of against it.

Chapter Six

Everyone Needs Me and I Have Nothing Left

How to protect your energy without disappearing from your life

Natalie thought she was doing everything "right." She'd done the biology work. She'd gotten more clarity. She was trying to be disciplined and grateful and hydrated-because apparently adulthood is just carrying a water bottle and acting calm while your brain quietly runs sixteen tabs in the background.

Then it happened again: a small request at home hit her at the wrong moment and she snapped. Not dramatic. Just sharp enough to sting. Then guilt arrived immediately, like it had been waiting in the hallway with its shoes on.

The thought she couldn't shake was this: Everyone needs me and I have nothing left. If that sentence feels familiar, hear this first: you are not alone. Midlife can create a perfect storm-hormonal shifts, sleep disruption, caregiving, identity changes, and relationship strain-all at once.

Your capacity doesn't shrink because you're weak. It shrinks because you're carrying more load with fewer reserves.

Why this area of work comes next

Area of Work #2 is Care-Focused Connection. It comes after Area #1 because once your biology starts to stabilize, the next bottleneck often isn't another lab or protocol-it's relational load: the people, obligations, transitions, and emotional labor that drain you even when your sleep and symptoms are improving. This is the move that turns frustration into flow because you stop living on accidental overdraft and start managing your energy like the real resource it is.

Your oxygen mask first, then everyone else

You know the airplane safety briefing: put your own oxygen mask on first, then help others. That isn't selfish. It's physics. If you're gasping, you don't become more helpful by trying harder-you become more frantic.

Midlife works the same way. When you're depleted, you don't become more loving by pushing through. You become more reactive. Protecting recovery isn't a luxury-it's oxygen. It's how you show up with patience instead of resentment.

This chapter is how you put the oxygen mask on-without disappearing from your life or turning every relationship into a negotiation.

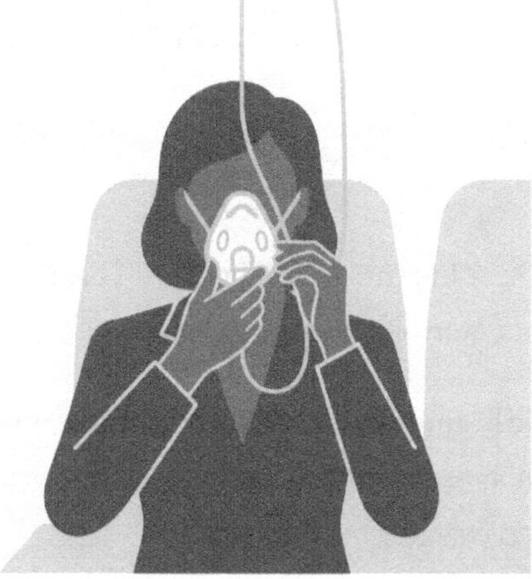

Step 1: The Social Energy Audit (7 days, no drama)

Natalie's breakthrough didn't come from a bigger plan. It came from a smaller one: stop guessing.

For one week, she did a quick check before and after the interactions that make up real life:

- Before: energy (1–10)
- After: energy (1–10)
- Label the energy use: Giver / Neutral / Drain / Vampire

A quick note so this stays kind (and funny, because we're not turning into robots): "'Vampire' isn't a character judgment-it's a cost category. Some situations are just... expensive." You are not diagnosing people. You're measuring cost-including the cost that shows up the next day, not just the cost you feel in the moment.

The story: Sunday lunch and the 48-hour hangover

On Sunday, Natalie did what she always did: lunch with her parents. It wasn't a disaster. No blow-ups. No scandal. Just normal-the kind of normal that looks perfectly fine... and then quietly takes you out on Tuesday.

- She walked in at a 6/10 and left at a 2/10. She wrote it down and moved on.
- Monday: she woke up heavy. Not sad-just slower, like her brain was loading on dial-up.
- Tuesday: same. Thin patience. Short fuse. That feeling of "I'm doing my best and I still want everyone to stop talking."

That's when she circled her note and finally told the truth: Sunday lunch = 48-hour drain. Not because her parents are villains. Not because she's fragile. Because the recovery cost is real-and her body was charging her interest.

Then she noticed something that made her laugh, because it was irritatingly true. On Wednesday, she took a 20-minute walk alone-no errands, no multitasking, no "I'll just answer one email while I'm breathing." She left at a 3/10 and came back at a 6/10. Meanwhile Netflix-who keeps promising "rest"-had been leaving her more tired, somehow still watching, and oddly invested in a show she doesn't even like. (She was still asking, "Do we really need another episode?" like the TV was pressuring her.)

That's the moment the thesis becomes real: she stops spending energy by accident and starts spending it on purpose. That's flow.

What to do with the data (so the audit actually changes your life)

Once you spot a 24–48–72-hour drain, you don't "power through" it-you adjust the plan. You change one of three levers:

- Time: shorter
- Frequency: less often
- Recovery: scheduled on purpose

The goal isn't to avoid your life. It's to stop paying for one "normal" event with three days of irritability.

Step 2: Boundaries that feel loving (not harsh)—the CLEAR Framework

Natalie didn't cancel her parents. She didn't announce a new identity. She didn't make a speech. She used CLEAR-a framework built for real life:

- C—Communicate early (before resentment builds)
- L—Lead with care (start from the relationship, not the rule)
- E—Explain your need (one sentence, no over-justification)
- A—Ask for what you need specifically (vague requests get vague responses)
- R—Reinforce if needed (boundaries often need restating—that is normal, not failure)

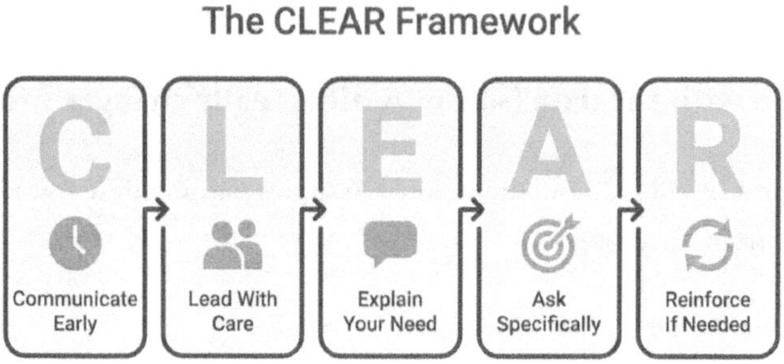

Two scripts you can borrow immediately:

"I need to check my energy levels before committing to that."

"I'm not available for calls after 8 PM-that's my recharge time."

Here's the part most women miss: respecting your limit means acting while you still look fine. If you wait until you're frantic, you end up setting boundaries with fire instead of clarity.

When Natalie made one calm adjustment-shorter time, more recovery-the next Sunday didn't disappear, but the two-day crash started to. Not perfect. Just better. Better enough that her irritability began to lift, and she felt something she hadn't felt in a while: permission.

Another version of the same problem: empty nest + relationship flatness

Care-Focused Connection isn't only for the "too many people need me" season. Sometimes it's for the quiet season-the one that surprises you.

Natalie didn't expect the empty nest to feel like grief. She thought it would feel like freedom. Instead, the house got quiet in a way that made her reorganize a drawer she doesn't even like-just to feel useful.

It wasn't that she missed the chaos-she missed being needed.

Her relationship didn't look broken. It looked... flat. Two adults sharing a Wi-Fi plan and occasionally asking, "Did you pay that bill?" They weren't fighting. They were just slowly disappearing from each other's daily life. Then the caregiving text arrives. The paperwork. The appointment. The invisible "Can you handle this?" that lands on her shoulders. She loves her family. But she's tired.

Love and capacity are not the same thing-and midlife exposes the difference.

Then, there is the grief that nobody warns you about: the one that arrives not when something goes wrong, but when something goes right.

Your children grew up. They left. That was supposed to be the victory—the thing you worked toward for twenty years. It is victorious. Except now the house is quiet in a way that sounds less like peace and more like absence. The schedule that used to run you ragged now has open spaces you do not know how to fill without feeling guilty for having them.

Some women describe it as losing their job title without a retirement party. The role that organized their identity—the scheduling, the driving, the knowing where everyone was at all times—simply ends. What remains is a question most women were too busy to ask while the chaos was still running: who am I when I am not needed?

If your relationship feels flat during this season, it may not be broken. It may simply be exposed. When the shared project of raising children no longer occupies the center of the partnership, what remains is whatever you and your partner built underneath it—and for many couples, the honest answer is: we did not build much underneath it. We were too busy.

That is not a failure. It is an opportunity. But it requires you to notice it, name it, and decide what you want to build next—with the same intentionality you brought to raising the humans who just left.

So she applies the same sequence: audit the cost, adjust the plan, and build recovery into real life. That's how you stop feeling isolated and irritated at the same time-like you're alone, but also needed by everyone.

-

Step 3: Strategic connection (so you don't confuse isolation with recovery)

When women are depleted, they often swing between:

- overcommitting and crashing, or
- withdrawing and calling it "rest."

A simple middle path is the 5-3-1 Weekly Strategy:

- 5 micro-restoratives (ten minutes or less—a walk, tea alone, quiet before the day starts)
- 3 connection investments (interactions that fill you, not just ones you owe)
- 1 boundary protected (one "no," one limit honored, one ask redirected)

This gives you structure without making your social life another job. The 5-3-1 is not about building a perfect social circle. It is about making sure your week includes recovery, connection, and at least one moment where you chose yourself.

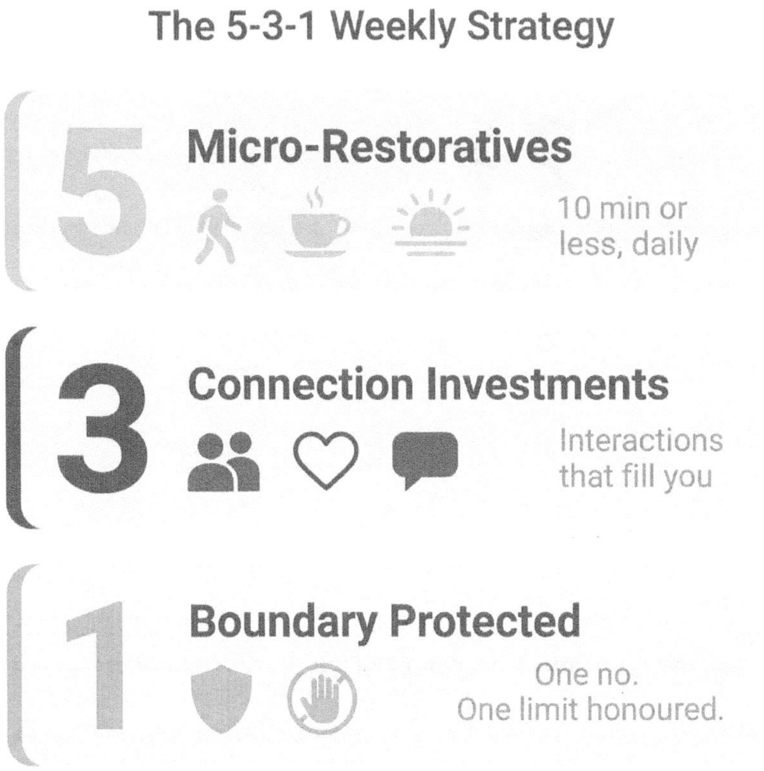

Step 4: Recovery that actually works—the 24-48-72 rule

Even "good" social weekends can be expensive in midlife. The solution isn't to stop living. It's to recover with intention.

The 24-48-72 Recovery Rule:

- 24 hours: gentle care (sleep, hydration, quiet, a walk)
- 48 hours: gradual re-entry (one thing, not five things)
- 72 hours: back to baseline

This is how you stop paying for one event with a full week of irritability.

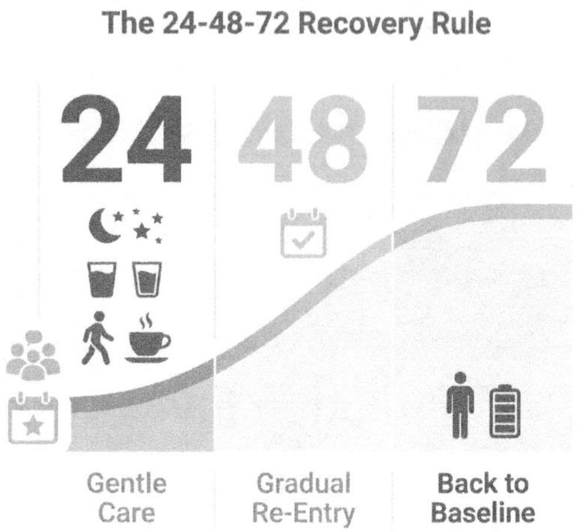

Here are the questions I hear most often – and the honest answers:

"Am I becoming antisocial?" No. You're becoming aware of capacity. Midlife can stack the deck. The goal isn't less life-it's smarter life.

"Why do I crash after something that was 'fine'?" Because "fine" isn't free. Some interactions include hidden work: managing tension, performing, hosting, caretaking. The audit reveals the recovery cost.

"Why do I snap at the people I love?" Often because home is where you stop performing. Many high-functioning women hold it together all day, then depletion shows up as irritability at night. That doesn't mean you're unloving. It means you're overdrawn.

"Is it selfish to protect my energy?" No. Your oxygen mask first, then everyone else. If you're gasping, no one wins. Protecting recovery is how you stay kind without resentment.

"What if people don't understand?" You don't need a committee vote. You need clear language and consistency. CLEAR helps you communicate early so boundaries don't come out as blow-ups later.

Your Week-One Mini Plan (three moves)

Move 1—Social Energy Audit (7 days). Rate energy before/after key interactions and label: Giver / Neutral / Drain / Vampire. Remember: "'Vampire' isn't a character judg-ment-it's a cost category. Some situations are just... expensive."

Move 2—Choose ONE CLEAR boundary. Pick the biggest drain the audit reveals. Change one lever: time, frequency, or recovery. Use one script:

- "I need to check my energy before committing."
- "I'm not available after 8 PM-that's my recharge time."

Move 3—Apply the 24-48-72 recovery rule. After an expensive event, plan recovery like it's part of the event. This is how you break the snap-guilt cycle. Optional add-on: sketch your 5-3-1 Weekly Strategy for the coming week. You are not failing at life. You are trying to live midlife without enough oxygen.

So here's the pivot-where frustration becomes flow: I will honor my energy needs without guilt. I will set boundaries that protect my wellbeing. I will choose connections that restore, not drain. I will build real recovery into my week. I will be patient with myself while I rebuild. Because the goal isn't to become someone new. It's to come back to yourself-without burning your life down to do it.

Your Chapter 6 Workbook Resource

The companion workbook turns this chapter into action. Scan the QR code below—or go to www.hotflashtohotdamnbook.com/workbook — to access the **Energy Audit**: a chapter-by-chapter look at where your energy is going and where the highest-return changes are waiting.

Chapter Seven

Off the Exam Table Paper

How to Walk Into Every Appointment Prepared and Finally Walk Out With the Care You Deserve

This chapter is about a room. Specifically, a room with a physician who has ten to fifteen minutes, a prescription pad within reach, and a system built for acute care—not for the complex, hormonal, layered experience you are living.

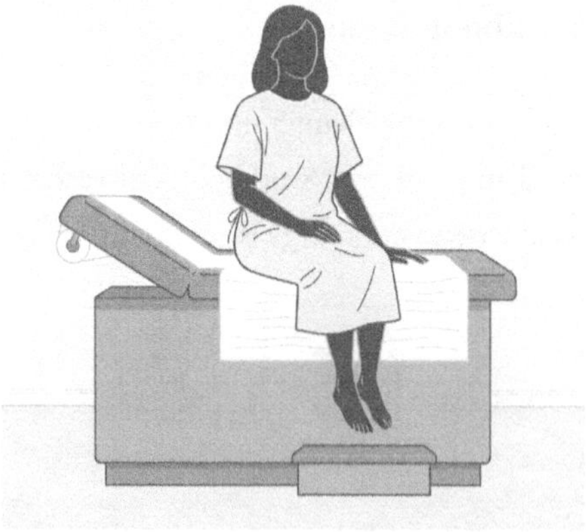

This is about how to prepare for it. How to speak inside it. How to walk out with something better than a prescription you didn't ask for and a quiet sense of defeat. If that room has ever made you feel small, you are not the problem—your strategy just needs an upgrade.

Natalie Returns

Natalie returns here—55, financial consultant, precise to her bones, and used to being the one with the answers. When her body started changing in ways she couldn't spreadsheet her way out of, she did what high performers do: she researched, tracked, tried harder... and ended up with more noise, not more clarity.

Now she's bringing what she's already learned in earlier chapters into the one place it has to work in real time: the exam room—where the clock is loud, the system is rushed, and she's done leaving with "you're fine" and a quiet sense of defeat.

Natalie's empty nest is newly quiet, her mother is in assisted living, and her body has been sending signals she can no longer explain away. Weight accumulating despite consistent effort. Joint aches every morning. Anxiety that shows up uninvited. Brain fog that makes her hesitate in meetings where she once felt sharp.

Natalie did what she always does when something isn't working: she researched. Podcasts, articles, lab results she found online, expert opinions. Instead of clarity, she got overwhelm. Every answer opened three more questions. She started doubting herself—not just physically, but intellectually. How could someone so capable feel so lost?

She walked into her third appointment in eight months with a color-coded folder, a two-page symptom summary, and forty-three minutes of information for a seven-minute appointment.

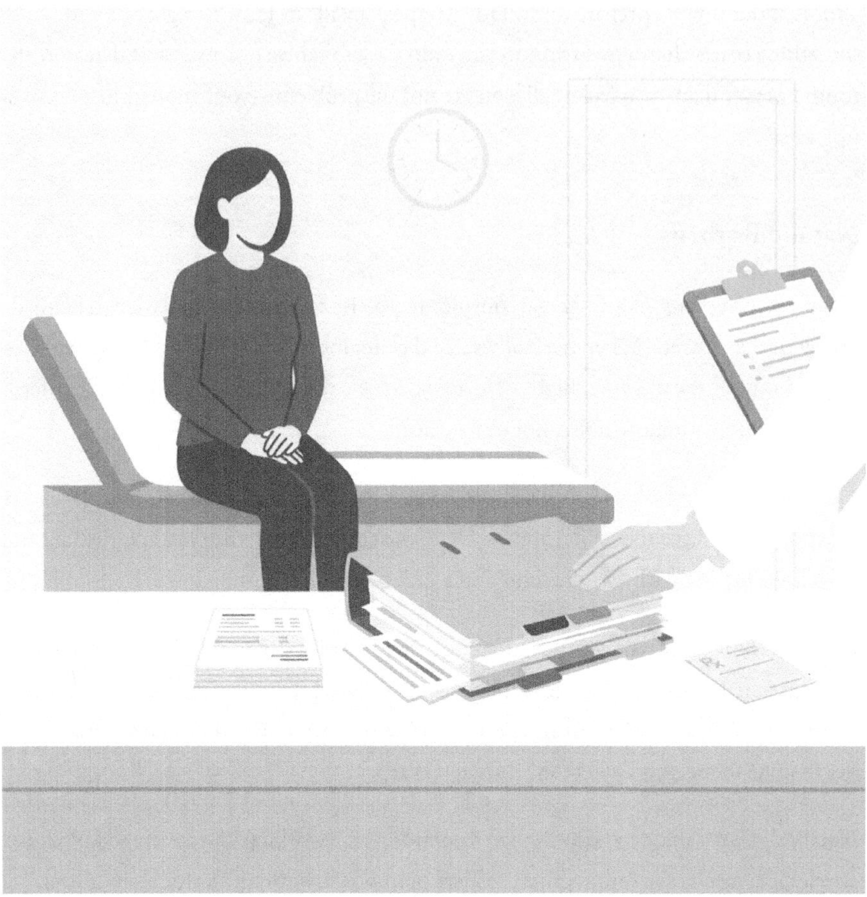

The physician—pleasant, visibly rushed—glanced at the folder, set it down, and said: "Your labs look fine."

Her brain went blank—the way it does when you realize you're about to leave with no plan again. Natalie felt the familiar tightening in her chest. Her questions sat unasked.

She left with a prescription for an antidepressant she had not asked for, no plan, and no follow-up scheduled. She didn't fill the prescription. She also didn't make another appointment for eleven months.

A note on the antidepressant

This is a common moment for midlife women—mood changes, anxiety, poor sleep, and fatigue get interpreted quickly, and an antidepressant gets offered early. Sometimes that medication is absolutely the right tool, and it can be life-changing. But it shouldn't be the only tool—or the automatic first stop—when there hasn't been a full evaluation of what else may be driving the change you're describing. If hormones, sleep disruption, nutrient issues, thyroid function, or chronic stress are part of the picture, you deserve a conversation that includes the full context—what's been checked, what hasn't, and what the plan is if this doesn't help.

The goal isn't to refuse help. The goal is to make sure you're getting the right help, in the right order, for the right reason.

What the Unprepared Appointment Actually Costs You

What happened to Natalie has a name. I call it "the everything-dump appointment"—and it is not a failure of intelligence. It is a structural mismatch. You arrive with everything. The system has room for almost nothing. It's not that you're too much. It's that the appointment is too small.

You walk out feeling not just unheard, but hopeless.

Hopelessness is a clinical outcome. When a woman stops believing the system can help her, she stops engaging with it. She delays care. She begins treating herself based on internet research—sometimes correctly, often without the clinical sequencing that keeps her safe. Or she cycles through provider after provider, collecting fragmented care with no one holding the full picture. The antidote is simple: leave every visit with a next step—a test, a referral, a trial, or a follow-up date.

There is also a quieter danger, especially for the high-performing woman: she gets labeled. A note in the chart that says "anxious," "demanding," or the word that follows a woman everywhere—"difficult"—travels with her into every future appointment. Electronic health records mean that label arrives before she does. It shapes how the next physician sees her before she says a word.

Documentation cuts both ways: it can carry labels forward, but it can also carry your clarity forward. That's why we're building a record that reflects your symptoms, your impact, and your plan—cleanly.

This is why how you communicate matters as much as what you say. It is not a soft skill. It is a clinical strategy. This is why we're going to get smart about communication—not to perform, but to get results.

The Shift That Makes Everything Else Work

Before tools and scripts, let's talk about something more important.

I have watched women with every resource available leave appointments empty-handed. I have watched women with a handwritten index card leave with exactly what they needed. The difference was never information. It was identity.

You bring a version of yourself into that exam room. For many high-performing women, that version is smaller than the one she brings everywhere else. At work, she negotiates, pushes back, asks for what she needs. In the exam room, she waits to be asked. She minimizes. She says, "I'm probably fine, I just wanted to check." She accepts the first answer, even when something in her knows it is not enough.

The shift this chapter asks of you is simple: let the capable version of you show up here, too. The woman who runs the meeting, who knows when a plan isn't working, who asks hard questions without apology—she already knows how to advocate. She just hasn't given herself permission to do it here.

I spent years on the other side of the exam table. As a physician, I understood the system's limitations better than most patients. Then I became the patient—after my breast cancer diagnosis, after medication induced menopause took my hormones overnight. I had the clinical knowledge.

What I had to find was the willingness to use it for myself.

You're the expert on your lived experience. Your clinician is the expert on medicine. A good appointment is what happens when both are allowed in the room.

The One Tool You Can Use Now: The Three-Goal Rule

If you only take one skill from this chapter, take this: the Three-Goal Rule. It turns a rushed visit into a structured conversation—and structure is where progress starts compounding.

Before every appointment—routine or urgent—identify three and only three goals:

- your primary concern,
- your secondary concern, and
- one preventive or follow-up item.

Write them down. Say them out loud at the start of the visit.

Here is why it works. It focuses you, it signals to your physician that you are organized and purposeful, and it turns an open-ended visit into a structured conversation. Physicians are trained to work within structure. Give it to them, and you get more in return.

A Three-Goal Statement sounds like this: "I have three things I'd like to cover today. My main concern is the fatigue and brain fog that have been affecting my work for the past four months. Second, I want to talk about my irregular cycles and the night sweats waking me up. Third, I'd like to discuss whether it's time for a bone density scan. Can we make sure we get to all three?"

Notice what that statement does. It is organized. It names the impact on daily life, not just the symptom. It includes a prevention question. It ends with a collaborative ask—not a demand, but an invitation.

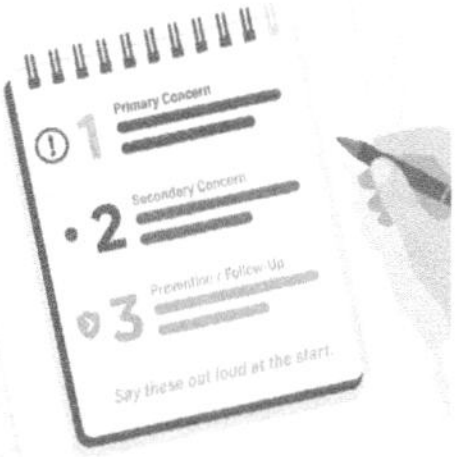

The Power Phrase: Assertive Without Adversarial

Here's the unfair truth: you may have three months of symptoms and 7-10 minutes of appointment time. The system was not built for what you're navigating. So rather than showing up with everything and hoping for the best, you're going to show up with clear priorities, one specific example of how your symptoms are affecting your life, and a defined next step you want before you leave. You can advocate fully and still speak in a way that gets traction—organized, direct, collaborative. That's not shrinking. That's working the room like the competent woman you already are. Unlike the exam table paper, it doesn't have to be uncomfortable.

The woman who says "I want you to order a full hormone panel" may be completely right. She may also walk out with nothing—because the request landed as a directive. The woman who says "I've been tracking my symptoms for six weeks and I'd love your input on what testing would give us the clearest picture" is asking for the same thing. But she has made her physician the expert and herself the informed partner. That framing costs nothing. It may change everything.

This is not about making yourself small. It is about being effective. There is a real difference between shrinking and being strategic.

Phrases That Open Doors

Instead of: "I need you to test my hormones." Try: "Given what I've been experiencing, what hormone testing would give us the most useful starting point?"

Instead of: "That's not good enough—I want more answers." Try: "I want to make sure we're not missing anything—what would you want to rule out before we settle on a plan?"

When a test or referral is declined: Try: "I understand. Could you document in my chart that I requested this and your reason for not ordering it? I want us both to have a clear record."

That last phrase is one of the most underused tools available to you. Asking a physician to document a declined request changes the dynamic in the room—not as a threat, but as calm, professional accountability. Many physicians will reconsider. Some will not. Either way, you now have information.

What a Good Appointment Looks Like

Eleven months later, Natalie walks in differently. She has done the work of this chapter. Three goals written down. Opening statement practiced in the car. A new physician, recommended by a friend who mentioned almost in passing: "She's current on menopause care—and she takes the whole picture seriously."

Natalie walks in prepared, not armored. She opens with her three goals. The physician listens—fully, without checking the clock. She asks questions. She connects Natalie's symptoms to the hormonal transition she is almost certainly moving through. She explains what the testing will show and why timing matters. She orders a full panel.

Then she does something that catches Natalie off guard: before Natalie leaves the office, the physician schedules a follow-up appointment to go over results and build a plan together. Natalie calls her sister on the drive home. "I think I finally found her."

This is the outcome. Not a miracle. Not an overnight cure. A physician who is current. A patient who feels heard. Testing that is appropriate and properly sequenced. A follow-up committed before she walked out the door.

That is the whole thing. That is where compounding begins.

The Appointment Upgrade (15 minutes)

Optional—if you want to level up results fast, this is the add-on.

Use this four-part structure before every medical appointment from here forward. It takes fifteen minutes. It will save you years of fragmented, frustrating care.

Step 1: Identify Your Three Goals. Write them, rank them, and name the impact—not just the symptom. "Brain fog" is a symptom. "Brain fog that caused me to miss critical details in a client meeting last week" is clinical communication.

Step 2: Bring One Data Point. Not seventeen. One. A recent lab result you have a question about. Three weeks of symptom notes. A summary of what you've already tried. Enough to show you're informed, not so much that it overwhelms the visit.

Step 3: Draft Your Power Phrase. Find the one thing you've never let yourself say. The ask you've swallowed. Write it down, reframe it as a collaborative question, and say it out loud before you walk in. Practice doesn't make perfect. Practice makes possible.

Step 4: Know Your Non-Negotiable. Decide before you go in: what does a successful appointment look like today? What is the one outcome you need? That clarity will keep you from leaving empty-handed—because you'll know the moment it's about to happen, and you'll have the words ready.

Your Action for Today

You don't need an appointment on the calendar to start. Do two things right now. First, write down your three goals for your next appointment—even if it's months away. Don't clean them up. Write what is actually true. What do you most need addressed? What have you been putting off? What have you been minimizing? Second, write down one power phrase you have never let yourself say to a doctor. Something you thought but swallowed. Reframe it as a collaborative ask using the language from this chapter, and then say it out loud—in your car, at your desk, wherever you are right now. These two acts start the compounding. Every appointment you navigate well builds skill, confidence, and a medical record that reflects who you actually are: a woman who knows her body, knows what she needs, and knows how to ask for it.

Your Chapter 7 Workbook Resources

The companion workbook turns this chapter into action. Scan the QR code below—or go to www.hotflashtohotdamnbook.com/workbook — to access the **Medical Advocacy Preparation Guide:** the exact questions to ask, the labs to request, and the language that gets you taken seriously in any clinical encounter.

Natalie found a better-fit physician and optimized her communication skills. You can, too—and even before you do, these skills help you get more out of every appointment. When you walk in ready, you don't show up as a patient hoping for help. You show up as a partner who knows what she needs and how to ask for it. That is not the end of the work. It is the beginning of the compounding.

Chapter Eight

It Wasn't You. It Was Your Biology

Not Willpower. Not Weakness. It Was Your Hormones All Along.

Advocacy gets you into the right room. But understanding your biology is what makes the results meaningful—what turns a lab panel into a roadmap. This chapter is about seeing yourself as a whole system, not a collection of separate symptoms, and building a plan that finally fits.

This is where the Precision Hormone Program you have been building since Chapter 1 arrives at its metabolic center. The Four-Layer Reset is not a separate system — it is the framework that explains why some women do everything right and still feel like their body is working against them. Cortisol first. Thyroid second. Hormones third. Metabolic support fourth. Every chapter that came before this one was clearing the path for exactly this sequence. Now we are going to walk it

There is something I want to be honest with you about before we go further. This book gives you the complete framework. The four layers, the cortisol reset, the thyroid piece, the hormone picture, the whole-woman approach—all of it is here. You can understand it, apply it, and begin to feel the difference. But hormone therapy decisions—the what, the when, the dose, the delivery method, the monitoring—require a physician who can read your specific labs, your personal history, and the particular way your biology is presenting right now. Not because you are not capable of understanding it. You clearly are. But because your biology is not generic, and neither should your protocol be. That is not a limitation of this book. It is a feature of your body. It is exactly why having the right clinical partner matters.

If you have spent years doing everything right and watching your body do everything wrong-this chapter is your vindication.

Natalie Gets Her Results

Remember Natalie? Fifty-five. Financial consultant. Precise, analytical, high-performing. The woman who drove home from her new physician's office saying, "I think I finally found her." Two weeks later, she is back. Her results are in. For the first time in years, someone is connecting the dots. Not with a single magic number-through a full picture: hormones that have shifted, metabolic markers that explain the weight resistance, a stress pattern that matches how long she's been running on high alert, and nutrient gaps that quietly drain recovery. Natalie isn't hearing, "You're fine." She's hearing, "This makes sense-and we can build a plan from here."

Natalie listens. Then she says the thing she has been holding for three years: "I go to the gym five days a week. I eat well-mostly. I keep telling myself I just need to try harder. I thought I was broken. Or lazy. Or both."

Her physician looks at her steadily. "You are not unmotivated or lazy. Your biology changed-and nobody explained it to you."

Natalie cries. Not from sadness. From relief.

That moment-when the self-blame lifts and the science steps in-is what this chapter is built around. You cannot build a plan from shame. But from understanding? You can build anything.

This Was Never a Willpower Problem

Midlife weight gain is not a discipline problem. It is a systems problem. The system that broke down was not your character-it was your biology.

The weight gain, the brain fog, the broken sleep, the anxiety that shows up uninvited, the belly that wasn't there before-these are not four separate problems. They are one story told by different systems responding to the same upstream conditions.

Here's the part no one says plainly enough: weight loss and body composition are a high-demand ask in midlife-not because you're undisciplined, but because you're asking your body to do something biologically expensive: burn stored fuel, build or keep muscle, regulate appetite, sleep well, and stay emotionally steady... all at the same time.

If your system is running on low sleep, high stress chemistry, shifting hormones, and inconsistent recovery, "eat less and move more" doesn't land like a plan-it lands like a fight. This is why so many women do everything "right" and feel like their body is doing everything "wrong." It's not sabotage. It's logistics.

So before we talk tactics, we need a map that shows how the foundations connect-because when you address them in sequence, your body stops resisting and starts cooperating.

Here's the bird's-eye view that makes the whole thing make sense.

The 4-Layer Midlife Reset (Bird's-Eye Map)

Not a program with a start and end date—a way of seeing yourself clearly, so your plan finally fits.

A note before we go further: this framework looks at weight and body composition specifically.

The hierarchy you learned in earlier chapters—cortisol first, thyroid second, sex hormones third—still holds. What this map adds is the recognition that when it comes to weight in midlife, there is a layer beneath cortisol that drives it: the psychosocial load that keeps cortisol elevated in the first place.

Your boundaries, your emotional labor, your chronic state of being needed by everyone—those are not soft factors. They are the upstream trigger for the stress chemistry that makes weight loss biologically expensive. That is why psychosocial regulation appears first here. It is not replacing the hormone hierarchy. It is naming what sits above it when weight is the lens.

Layer 1: Psychosocial Regulation (the "upstream trigger" layer)

Boundaries, self-advocacy, reducing chronic emotional load, and nervous system repair. This is where you stop living like you are on call for everyone else's life. When psychosocial load stays high, cortisol stays high—and everything downstream stalls. The work you did in Chapter 6 is not separate from weight management. It is the beginning of it.

The clinical evidence supports this sequence. Research published in *Obesity Reviews* (Tomiyama, 2019) demonstrates that chronic psychosocial stress independently predicts visceral fat accumulation in women, even after controlling for diet and exercise. A landmark study in *Psychoneuroendocrinology* (Epel et al., 2001) showed that women with the highest perceived stress had significantly higher cortisol reactivity, which was directly correlated with greater abdominal fat deposition. A 2022 meta-analysis in the *International Journal of Obesity* confirmed that psychological stress interventions produced meaningful reductions in waist circumference and visceral adiposity, independent of dietary change. In other words: addressing the psychosocial layer is not a soft recommendation. It is a clinically supported upstream intervention for the metabolic changes that make midlife weight loss feel impossible.

Layer 2: Cortisol stabilization (the "out of survival mode" layer)

Sleep restoration, recovery rhythms, and lowering chronic activation. When cortisol steadies, appetite steadies. Cravings quiet down. Your body becomes less defensive. This is the same cortisol-first work from Chapter 3—applied now to the specific question of why your body stores fat around the middle and refuses to let it go.

Layer 3: Thyroid and Hormone Optimization (the "terrain" layer)

Your thyroid sets the metabolic speed. Your sex hormones influence where fat is stored, how hunger signals behave, how well you keep muscle, and how deeply you sleep. When the thyroid is off—even subtly—the metabolic engine runs cold, and the same effort produces less result. When sex hormones are unsupported, the terrain shifts: hunger gets louder, fullness gets quieter, and fat settles more easily around the middle.

This is why Chapters 4 and 5 matter here. If your thyroid has not been fully evaluated, and your sex hormones have not been addressed as a connected system, this layer may be the reason everything else feels stuck.

Layer 4: Metabolic Support (the "engine" layer)

Strength training, protein-forward nutrition, rebuilding metabolic flexibility, and—when appropriate—medical tools like GLP-1 therapy as leverage, not a shortcut. This is where the body starts responding again because the engine is finally being supported instead of punished.

You do not need to do all four layers perfectly to see change. You just need to stop treating weight as an isolated problem and start treating it like what it is in midlife: a systems outcome. Address the upstream conditions, and the downstream results follow.

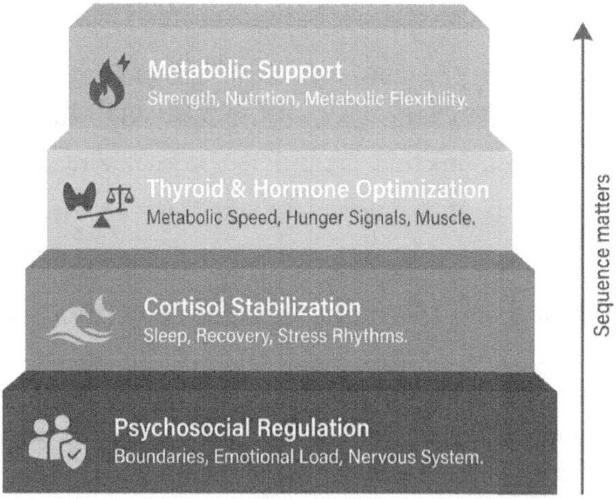

Layer 1: Psychosocial Regulation—The Part People Skip (and then wonder why nothing works)

This is where the reset begins—not at the gym, not at the pharmacy, but in the chronic emotional load your nervous system has been carrying without relief.

In earlier chapters we talked about the emotional labor of midlife-the caregiving, the career demands, the constant state of being needed by everyone except yourself. We talked about boundaries not as a lifestyle preference but as a biological necessity. Here is why that conversation matters physically.

Your body does not distinguish between caregiving stress, work stress, and financial stress. It just registers: we are under pressure.

When you live in constant pressure, you don't just feel tired. You become more reactive. You snack differently. You sleep differently. You recover differently. You make decisions differently. You end up blaming your "willpower" for what is really a capacity problem.

This is why boundaries and stress management are not soft skills. They are the beginning of biology cooperating again.

Layer 2: Cortisol Stabilization—The Quiet Driver

Once the emotional pressure starts to ease, the next job is getting cortisol out of the driver's seat. This layer is about sleep, recovery, and breaking the loop your body has been stuck in.

When pressure is sustained, cortisol-your primary stress hormone-stays elevated well past its welcome. Chronically high cortisol increases appetite, shifts fat storage toward the abdomen, makes blood sugar more unstable, makes muscle harder to keep, and breaks up sleep-which restarts the whole cycle the next morning.

This is the loop that makes women feel like their bodies are "stuck":

- You're stressed, so cortisol rises.
- Sleep gets fragmented.

- Your appetite signals get louder and less predictable.
- Energy dips, cravings rise, workouts feel harder, recovery gets worse.
- You compensate with caffeine and discipline.

Then you do it again tomorrow.

This is why "stress management" isn't a spa recommendation. It's metabolic medicine. When you protect your time and build recovery into your day, you are directly influencing your body's ability to manage weight.

Unmanaged stress almost guarantees resistance to change.

Layer 3: Hormone Optimization—More Than You Were Told

With stress chemistry settling and sleep improving, your hormonal environment becomes both more visible and more responsive. This is the layer where the clinical picture finally starts to make sense.

Most women are told estrogen regulates their menstrual cycle. True-but a fraction of the story. Estrogen also influences appetite and fullness signals in the brain, how the body distributes fat, how well it maintains muscle, sleep quality, insulin sensitivity, and mood. It is a whole-body regulating force.

As estrogen declines in perimenopause and menopause, hunger gets louder, fullness gets quieter, fat settles more easily around the middle, and muscle declines faster without active effort. This is why women say: "I am eating the same things, moving the same way-but my body is not the same."

They are right. No amount of willpower changes a shifted hormonal environment.

For the right person at the right time, bioidentical hormone therapy can improve sleep, ease hot flashes and night sweats, stabilize mood, and remove major obstacles to metabolic health.

Hormones are not a weight-loss treatment. But if you are waking at 2 a.m. drenched in sweat and running on caffeine by 7 a.m., you are not in a position to lose weight. When appropriate, hormonal support can reset the terrain so everything else can work.

A note from your author—who really should have known better

My body had been through a lot. After my breast cancer diagnosis and years on tamoxifen, my hormones didn't so much "transition" as get quietly escorted off the stage-clinically indicated, personally inconvenient.

I was a physician. I knew the physiology. I could explain the mechanism in my sleep. Yet I still gained 45 pounds in three years while going to the gym five or six days a week and eating what I'd generously describe as "mostly well," with occasional lapses involving a cheese board and zero regret.

I did a lot of things right. My body had other plans.

I've since rebuilt-with strength training, a protein-forward diet, imperfect stress management between a busy practice and adult children with a talent for appearing at dinnertime-and yes, a low-dose GLP-1 as part of a comprehensive plan.

If a physician who teaches this material couldn't outwork her own biology, neither could you. Neither of you should have had to.

Which brings us to the next layer: when stress and hormone shifts pile up, the place it often shows up first is in your metabolism-how your body handles energy, hunger, and fat storage.

Layer 4: Metabolic Support—Where It All Lands

The first three layers create the conditions. This layer is where your metabolism—your body's ability to use energy efficiently—finally gets to do its job again.

Cortisol and estrogen shifts set the stage. Metabolic inflexibility is where the story lands.

Think of your metabolism like a hybrid car. When it's working well, it switches smoothly between burning carbohydrates and burning fat, energy stays stable, and the engine runs cleanly. When that flexibility is lost, you get stuck running on one fuel-usually sugar-and when it dips, everything crashes. Hunger hits hard. Energy drops. Fat around the abdomen stops responding to what used to work.

Menopause is associated with a real and measurable loss of this metabolic flexibility. Add chronic stress and poor sleep, and the loss accelerates. This is why short periods without eating feel harder than they used to. Why your thirties strategies produce nothing in your fifties.

But metabolic inflexibility is not permanent. It is a downstream result of everything upstream. Address the upstream conditions-stress, hormones, sleep-and metabolic flexibility begins to return.

The system starts working with you again.

The Protein-Forward Mediterranean Framework (a quick reference)

The nutritional approach that supports all four layers is simpler than most programs make it: a Mediterranean-style foundation built around adequate protein, healthy fats, vegetables, and whole grains—with protein as the anchor, not the afterthought. In midlife, protein requirements increase, and most women are not eating enough to protect muscle, support hormone production, and stabilize blood sugar. A reasonable starting target is approximately one gram of protein per pound of ideal body weight daily, spread across meals. Build each plate around a quality protein source, add colorful vegetables, include healthy fats (olive oil, avocado, nuts), and let whole grains play a supporting role rather than the starring one. This is not a diet. It is a framework—flexible enough to fit your life and consistent enough to change your biology.

Why This Is About More Than the Scale

There is nothing wrong with wanting to feel comfortable in your clothes again, or to look in a dressing room mirror without dreading it. Those desires are real and valid. This chapter does not ask you to apologize for them.

But the stakes are larger. The fat that accumulates around the abdomen and internal organs during menopause is not inert. It produces inflammatory signals. Chronic low-grade inflammation is a primary driver of heart disease, stroke, type 2 diabetes, cognitive decline, and accelerated aging.

When we improve blood sugar control, reduce this type of fat, build muscle, regulate stress, sleep better, and support hormones-when appropriate-we are not just changing how you look. We are changing your trajectory.

Weight loss becomes the doorway. A longer, stronger, sharper life is the destination.

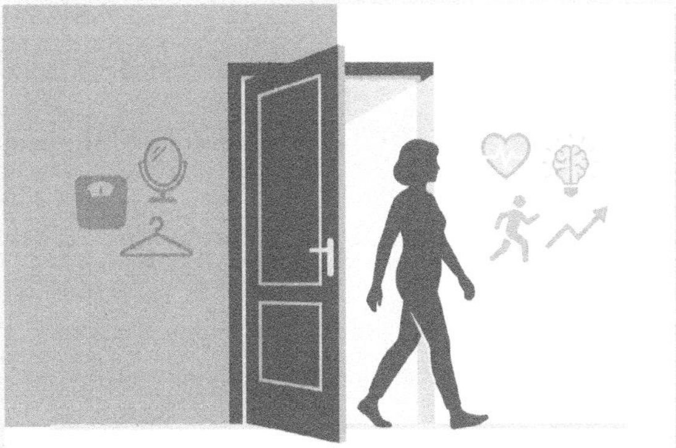

Weight loss is the doorway. Longevity is the destination.

A Word on GLP-1 Therapy: Leverage, Not a Shortcut

You've heard about GLP-1 medications. The attention has been enormous-and the conversation is often either a hype train or a moral debate. I'm not interested in either.

Here's the simple truth: GLP-1 is a hormone your body already makes. It helps with fullness after eating, slows stomach emptying, improves insulin response, and quiets the relentless appetite noise that can make every food decision feel like a negotiation.

For some women in midlife-especially when sleep is disrupted, stress is high, hormones have shifted, and weight has become stubborn-GLP-1 therapy can create enough breathing room for the rest of the plan to finally work.

But here's the non-negotiable: medication alone is not transformation. It is leverage. The foundation still matters-strength training to protect muscle, adequate protein, sleep, stress regulation, and hormone support when appropriate. If those pieces aren't in place, you can lose weight and still feel worse, look more tired, or end up right back where you started.

The goal is not "thin at any cost." The goal is better biology: improved metabolic health, preserved muscle, steadier energy, and a body that responds again.

Because this is medicine – not a trend – GLP-1 decisions should be made with a qualified clinician who can review your full history, monitor side effects, and adjust the plan over time. This is shared decision-making, not a one-size-fits-all prescription.

If you want to explore whether this is right for you, bring it to your next appointment using the language from Chapter 7: "Given my metabolic picture, am I a candidate for GLP-1 therapy as part of a comprehensive plan?"

That framing shows you understand it is one tool-not the whole answer.

What Working With You Actually Feels Like

Six weeks later, Natalie is working through all four layers. Not perfectly-nobody does. She cancelled her gym session twice, had a week where stress ate her sleep routine alive, and is still negotiating with herself about the 10 p.m. snacking habit she's had since her kids were teenagers.

But something has shifted.

Last Tuesday she put on a pair of trousers she had quietly moved to the back of the closet eight months ago. They buttoned. Not comfortably-but they buttoned. She stood in her bedroom and felt something she had almost forgotten: her body responding.

The following Saturday she went clothes shopping-something she had avoided for over a year. In the fitting room, under fluorescent lights that are unkind to everyone, she tried on three things. Two of them fit. She did not hate the mirror.

That is the moment. Not a dramatic transformation. Trousers that button. A fitting room that doesn't ruin the afternoon. A body beginning, finally, to work with her.

It started because she stopped treating herself as a list of problems and started treating herself as a system that needed the right conditions. The shame stopped. The strategy started. Everything else compounded from there.

Your Action for Today: Just One Thing

I am not asking you to overhaul your life today. I know what you are already carrying. Scan the QR code below to open your Chapter 8 workbook. Find the 4-Layer Reset Checklist. Read through all four layers. Then pick one thing-one single action from any layer that feels manageable right now. Not the hardest thing. The one thing that, when you do it, signals to your body and your mind that the reclamation has begun.

One thing. That is the whole assignment. Everything else compounds from there.

Your Chapter 8 Workbook Resources

The companion workbook turns this chapter into action. Scan the QR code below—or go to www.hotflashtohotdamnbook.com/workbook — to access the **4-Layer Reset Checklist**: your personalized implementation tool for framework in this chapter, with space to identify your starting point in each layer.

Area of Work #3: Elevation

Done surviving. Time to design the next decade.

The four layers you built in the last chapter are your foundation—the conditions that had to stabilize before elevation was possible. What follows is what you build on that foundation. Some of it will look familiar: strength training, nutrition, sleep. The difference is the intention. You are no longer stabilizing. You are building. You are no longer recovering from midlife. You are designing what comes next.

Chapter Nine

Done Surviving. Time to Thrive

From Restoration to Elevation — Becoming the Architect of Your Own Health

The Four-Layer Reset stabilized your foundation. What follows is what you build on it. The Six Pillars of Elevation are not a replacement for what came before — they are the next level of the same Precision Hormone Program, applied now to a body that is finally ready to respond. You are not starting over. You are moving up. There is a meaningful difference between a woman who is managing her biology and a woman who is designing her decade. This chapter is where that shift happens.

I want to tell you where I am right now.

Not where I was – the breast cancer, the tamoxifen, the 45 pounds, the gym sessions that produced nothing. You know that part. I want to tell you about an ordinary Tuesday morning, because that is the part that matters for what comes next.

I wake up without an alarm. I have a full practice, adult children who appear at dinnertime with the reliability of a natural phenomenon, and a life that has not slowed down for my wellness plan. I wake up because my body is ready. I take my supplements without negotiating. I train three to four times a week and protect those sessions the way I protect my most important patient commitments. I am not perfect. But I am consistent.

Turns out the secret isn't a secret-it's repetition. Which is both inspiring and deeply annoying.

Here's what I learned the hard way: I did not get here by recovering. I got here by deciding that recovery was not the destination. Recovery was just the doorway.

Everything you've done in the previous chapters-the mindset work, the advocacy, the biological understanding, the four-layer framework-that was restoration. Essential. You can't build on a cracked foundation. But the foundation is solid now. What comes next is elevation: the part where you stop recovering from midlife and start designing the next decade on purpose.

The Inflection Point

There is a moment in every woman's health journey where the path forks.

On one side: the comfortable plateau-feeling better than before, functional, grateful. On the other side: the decision to become an active architect of the next decade of your life.

You are standing at that fork right now.

If you choose to pause here, that's not failure. But it helps to know what's true: your body keeps aging whether you're intentional about it or not. The difference is that now you have leverage.

Strength, sleep, and muscle aren't "nice to have" in the second half of life-they're the infrastructure.

You've probably seen what happens when women don't get support, don't get education, and don't get a plan. They're not weak-they're under-resourced. They're doing their best inside a system that told them to "just deal with it." This chapter is your off-ramp.

The women who thrive in their sixties and beyond aren't superhuman. They're just the ones who stopped treating health like a crisis response. They picked a few non-negotiables, repeated them long enough to matter, and let the results stack.

Boring? Sometimes.

Effective? Always.

The Blaze of Glory Approach to Aging

I have a philosophy I share with my patients and anyone else who will listen: I refuse to go quietly into the night. I plan to burn out in a blaze of glory.

Not recklessly-in the best possible way. Fully alive, engaged, and present for as long as I am here. This is a quiet rebellion against the idea that midlife means decline. It does not. Midlife is recalibration. The women who understand that have a real advantage.

Also, to be clear: "blaze of glory" is not code for "run yourself into the ground." I am not trying to win the Olympic event of Exhaustion. I'm trying to stay strong enough to enjoy my life while I'm living it.

When I train consistently, I am a better physician, a more patient parent, a better partner. When my sleep is protected, my thinking is sharper.

When my hormones are supported and my nutrition is intentional, the woman in the mirror looks the way I feel inside-and that alignment between inner health and outer appearance is something I had lost for years without fully realizing what it cost me.

You do not have to earn the right to feel attractive, energetic, and confident in the second half of your life.

You just have to decide to pursue it. Then do the work.

Natalie Decides

Natalie has been working her four-layer plan for three months. The trousers button comfortably now. Sleep is reliably better. She has started strength training twice a week and, with some surprise, looks forward to it.

She feels better – genuinely, measurably better. Still, she senses she is hovering at the edge of something larger. She's using the map-and it's working. Which is exactly why the next question shows up: if you can feel better... how much better do you want to feel?

At her next appointment, her physician asks the question that changes everything: "You have done the hard part. Now I want to ask you something different. Not what you want to fix-what do you want your life to feel like in ten years?"

Natalie is quiet. Then: "I want to look like I feel. I want to be sharp. I want energy for what matters. I want to be someone my kids point to and say-she figured it out."

That is the inflection point. Not the first supplement. Not the first workout. The moment she stopped asking "How do I fix this?" and started asking "What do I want to build?"

That is when recovery ends and elevation begins.

The Six Pillars of Elevation

Area of Work #3 is built on six pillars. All matter. All are ultimately necessary. But you do not have to master them today-you just have to begin.

We're not doing this like a checklist.

We're going to do it like those "choose your own adventure" books we read as kids-except instead of fighting dragons, you're fighting the modern villain: inconsistency.

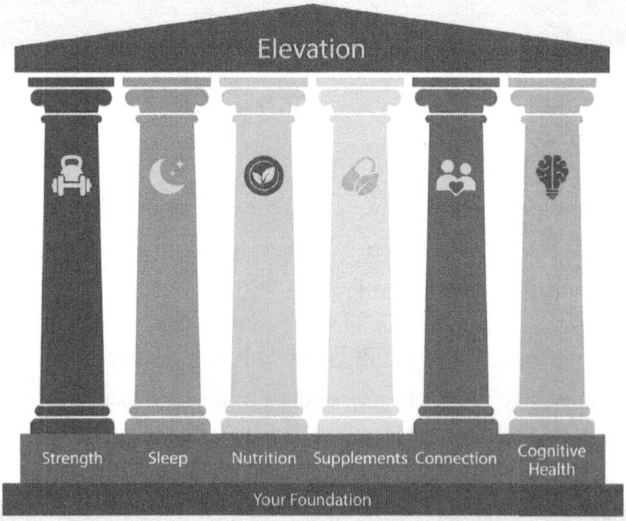

Step 1: Choose Your Anchor (pick ONE). These are the two fastest ways to change how you feel day-to-day: Anchor Option A: Strength Training and Muscle Preservation Muscle is your metabolic engine. It keeps your body burning fuel efficiently, protects your joints, supports bone density, and is one of the strongest predictors of longevity we have. When you train with resistance consistently, you feel capable in your body in a way that radiates quiet confidence. Two to three sessions a week. Even twenty minutes shifts the trajectory.

Anchor Option B: Sleep as a Non-Negotiable. Sleep is where your brain repairs, your hormones reset, and your skin regenerates. It is one of the most powerful anti-aging tools available-at zero cost. When it is protected, mood stabilizes, appetite regulates, and the face in the morning looks rested rather than worn. Guard it the way you guard your most important commitments.

Pick one. Anchor it. Repeat it.

Step 2: Add the Second Anchor (the one you didn't pick). If you chose strength training first, sleep becomes the support beam that makes training work. If you chose sleep first, strength training becomes the engine that makes the body respond. This is the "two-pillar base" that stops you from getting stuck in the cycle of: I'm trying so hard, why isn't this moving?

Step 3: Nutrition That Works With Your Biology. Every meal either supports or disrupts your hormonal environment, your inflammation levels, and your metabolic health. A Mediterranean-style diet built around clean protein, healthy fats, and vegetables gives your body the raw materials for everything else on this list. Investing in quality food is one of the highest-return decisions you can make.

In midlife, nutrition isn't just "eat clean." It's "eat enough of the right things so your body stops acting like you're in a famine."

Step 4: Strategic Supplementation. Even a well-designed diet leaves gaps-and midlife creates specific needs food alone cannot always meet. Targeted supplements can support energy, hormonal balance, brain function, and skin health. The goal is a clean, evidence-based approach matched to your biology.

All supplement decisions should be made with your healthcare provider. The workbook includes a clinical framework to start that conversation-without walking into your appointment sounding like you got your medical degree from a comment section.

Step 5: Social Connection and Purpose. Loneliness isn't just a mood-it has real effects on stress hormones, inflammation, sleep, and long-term health. The women who do best long-term tend to have steady relationships and a sense that their presence matters. Purpose isn't fluff. It's physiology.

If you lost yours in the caregiving years, this is your invitation to find it again.

Step 6: Cognitive Health and Mental Engagement. Your brain responds to exercise, nutrition, sleep, hormones, and connection the way your muscles do: it adapts to what you repeatedly ask of it. Staying sharp isn't about doing crossword puzzles out of fear. It is about staying genuinely curious, challenged, and purposeful. The woman who has that radiates something unmistakable.

The Question That Changes Everything

Information alone does not create change. What creates lasting change is finding something inside yourself that genuinely wants the outcome-not because you were told to, but because it is yours.

This is the core of motivational interviewing-one of the most evidence-based approaches to behavior change we have. Change that comes from within is change that lasts. You are not looking for the goal that looks most impressive. You are looking for the one that makes something inside you lean forward when you imagine it.

Sit with these questions. Write your answers if it helps. There are no right answers-only honest ones.

- When you imagine yourself one year from now, fully committed to your health-what does your daily life feel like?
- Which of the six pillars, if it were working well, would make the biggest difference to how you feel each day?
- What has it already cost you to not prioritize this-not in blame, but in honest

acknowledgment?

- What is one step in any pillar that feels genuinely possible this week-not the most impressive, the most real?
- What would it mean to you-your relationships, your work, your sense of self-if you actually did this?

The answer to question four is your action for today. Not mine. Yours.

What Becomes Possible

Let me paint you a picture-not a fantasy, but a realistic, achievable picture of what life looks and feels like when these pillars are active.

- You wake up rested. Your mind is clear from the first moment. You have energy that holds through the day without crashing at 3 p.m. You feel steady-emotionally, physically, hormonally-and you still have something left for the people and things that matter most.
- You look in the mirror and recognize the person looking back. Not your twenty-five-year-old self-something better. A woman who has lived through real difficulty and come out the other side with her health intact and her vitality growing.
- The glow you see is not makeup. It is the outward sign of a body that is genuinely well-balanced, nourished, rested, and strong.
- You feel confident and attractive in a way that has nothing to do with a number on a scale. It comes from knowing you are investing in yourself-not being carried by the current, but swimming through it with intention.
- The benefits spill into everything. Relationships improve. Work sharpens. Patience deepens. You become the woman whose energy other people feel-not because you are performing vitality, but because you are living it.

This is not the beginning of your decline. This is the beginning of your most powerful chapter yet.

Your Action for Today

Scan the QR code below to open your Chapter 9 workbook. Inside is the Healthspan Audit-a self-assessment across all six pillars that shows you clearly where you are doing well, where there is room to grow, and where your best first step might be.

Complete it honestly. Then sit with question four. Find the step that feels real-not the most impressive one, the one that genuinely calls to you. That is the one that will happen. That is the one that starts the compounding.

There are excellent practitioners in your area who can support this journey-physicians, nutritionists, trainers, and coaches who specialize in exactly what you are navigating. You do not have to do this alone. Asking for support is not weakness. It is strategy.

You have everything you need to begin. The tools are in your hands. The knowledge is in your head. The motivation, if you have been honest with yourself above, is already inside you. It always was.

Your Chapter 9 Workbook Resource

The companion workbook turns this chapter into action. Scan the QR code below—or go to www.hotflashtohotdamnbook.com/workbook — to access the **6-Pillar Healthspan Audit**: a clear-eyed assessment of where you are across all six pillars and which one deserves your attention first.

Natalie drove home from that appointment without putting on a podcast. She drove in silence, thinking about what her life could feel like in ten years if she actually did this. By the time she pulled into her driveway, she had made a decision. Not a list. Not a plan. A decision.

She was done drifting. She was ready to build.

The outside catching up to the inside.

You have rebuilt the foundation. You have stabilized the biology, protected your energy, advocated for your care, and started building the life you actually want. You have done the inside work. Now it is time to let the outside finally catch up. What follows is the part nobody talks about in hormone books: the moment when your outside finally starts telling the same story as your inside. These chapters are not about vanity. They are about congruence. They are about looking in the mirror and recognizing the woman you have become.

Chapter Ten

Damn Girl, You Got This!

Image Alignment — When the Outside Finally Catches Up to the Inside

There was a Tuesday morning—nothing special about it. My hair doing exactly what it had been doing since my hyperthyroidism took most of it, the cats unimpressed, the coffee not yet finished.

I caught my reflection. And stopped.

Not because everything was perfect. It wasn't. But something had settled. For the first time in longer than I wanted to admit, the woman looking back didn't feel foreign. Not completely herself again—but no longer lost either.

That shift didn't come from a serum.

What built it was everything underneath – the cortisol work, the thyroid finally taken seriously, hormones addressed as a connected system. The boundaries. The sleep. The strength training I had spent two years negotiating my way out of before reluctantly showing up for it.

All of it, in the right order, had been quietly doing its work. For the first time in a long time, what I saw matched what I felt.

You have done that work. Nine chapters of it. Something has shifted—in your energy, your resilience, the way you move through a hard day without the old empty arriving right behind it.

But here is what I want to ask you honestly: when you look in the mirror, does what you see match how you feel?

For many women, even after all the inside work is done, the answer is still *not quite.* The skin tells a story you are no longer living. The face reflects years of cortisol and disrupted sleep and a body that was running on fumes for longer than it should have been. There is a quiet gap—not dramatic, not devastating, but present—between the woman you have become and the woman looking back at you.

Closing that gap is not vanity. It is the last layer of the work. It is exactly what this chapter is for. Not skincare as a product category. Not anti-aging as a battle.

This is about image alignment—the moment the outside finally tells the same story as the inside. You have done the hormone work, the sleep, the strength training, the nutrition, the purpose. You have earned the right to see it reflected back at you. Wanting to look good is not shallow. Feeling attractive and confident in your own skin has real effects on your relationships, your professional presence, your mental health, and your joy. You are allowed to want this. You deserve it.

Why I Stopped Looking

When my children were small, I was exhausted. When they were tweens and not yet driving, I was the chauffeur—working, cooking, doing laundry—and I was exhausted. When they became adults with adult-sized problems, I was still the one holding the net. Then parents started aging too, sometimes with devastating speed. Work didn't pause for any of it. In that context, skincare felt indulgent. Caring about how I looked—actually admitting it mattered—felt dangerously close to "vanity," which was the one thing a woman stretched across a dozen responsibilities could not afford to be accused of. So it got pushed aside. Along with everything else that was purely for me. Here's the thing: those caregiving years were also years my skin needed more support. Because underneath all the busyness, my hormones were shifting. My skin was paying attention.

Your Skin Has Been Listening to Your Hormones

Skin isn't just a surface concern. It's a living organ that responds to what's happening inside the body. Shifts in estrogen, stress load, sleep quality, and thyroid function can show up on the skin—sometimes before we can fully explain what feels "off."

Estrogen is one of skin's closest allies. It supports collagen, skin thickness, elasticity, and the moisture barrier. As estrogen declines in perimenopause and menopause, changes can feel fast: skin may become drier, thinner-looking, less bouncy. Fine lines can look more obvious. Pigment changes can stand out more. It often happens sooner than we expect—and it can feel personal, even though it isn't.

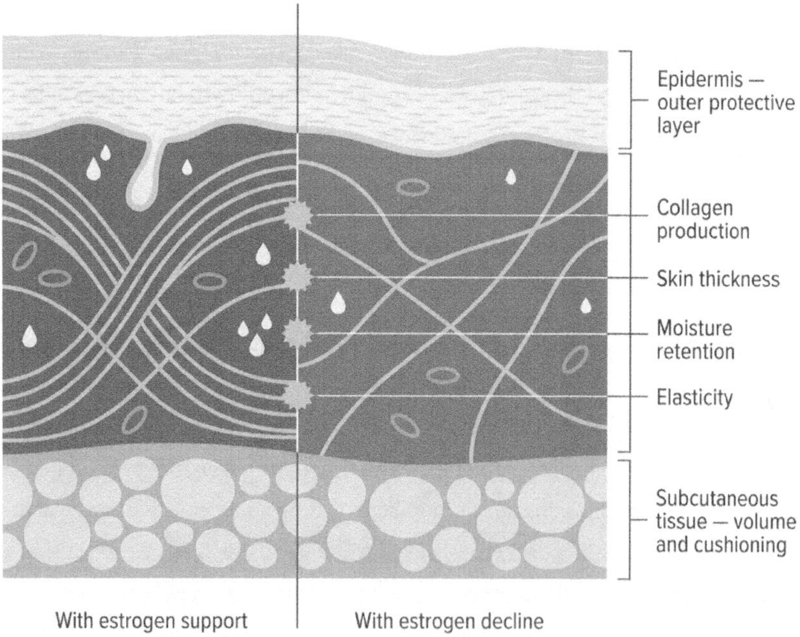

Chronic stress adds fuel to the fire. Long stretches of high stress can increase inflammation, slow repair, and disrupt sleep—when much of skin recovery happens. Stressed skin and hormonally shifting skin aren't the exact same problem, but they can stack together in a way that shows up clearly on the face.

This is why the work in the previous chapters is not separate from what we're discussing now. Optimizing hormones, stabilizing stress patterns, protecting sleep, building nutrition—all of that has already changed skin from the inside. The practice we're about to discuss is the amplifier. The internal work is the signal.

The Mirror Does Not Lie

I want to tell you about a moment in my own mirror. It was during the chaos that followed my breast cancer diagnosis—the tamoxifen, the hormonal disruption, the weight shift, and the stress of managing a life-altering diagnosis while still showing up to the world like everything was fine. I would stand at the mirror in the morning and smile. Something close to a real smile. But I could see that I wasn't right. The face looking back was telling a different story than the one I was performing for everyone else. It wasn't dramatic. It was a quiet wrongness I couldn't name, but couldn't stop noticing. I want to say this out loud because I think many women know exactly what I'm describing—and have never heard anyone admit it.

Seeing the evidence of what your body has been through written on your face can feel unsettling in a way that goes beyond vanity. It's a reminder that life is precious and finite. That the sand in the hourglass is real. That the woman in the mirror deserves to be genuinely cared for—not fixed or corrected, but tended to with the same intention she brings to everyone else.

The improvement, when it came, was a whisper. Slow, over months. The hormone work, the nutrition, the sleep, the supplements, the daily sunscreen I finally committed to. Then one ordinary Tuesday—nothing special about the day, my hair doing exactly what it has been doing since my hyperthyroidism took most of it—I looked in the mirror and thought: *Damn girl, you got this.* Nothing was perfect. But everything matched. I stopped bracing and just looked. That's what we're building toward.

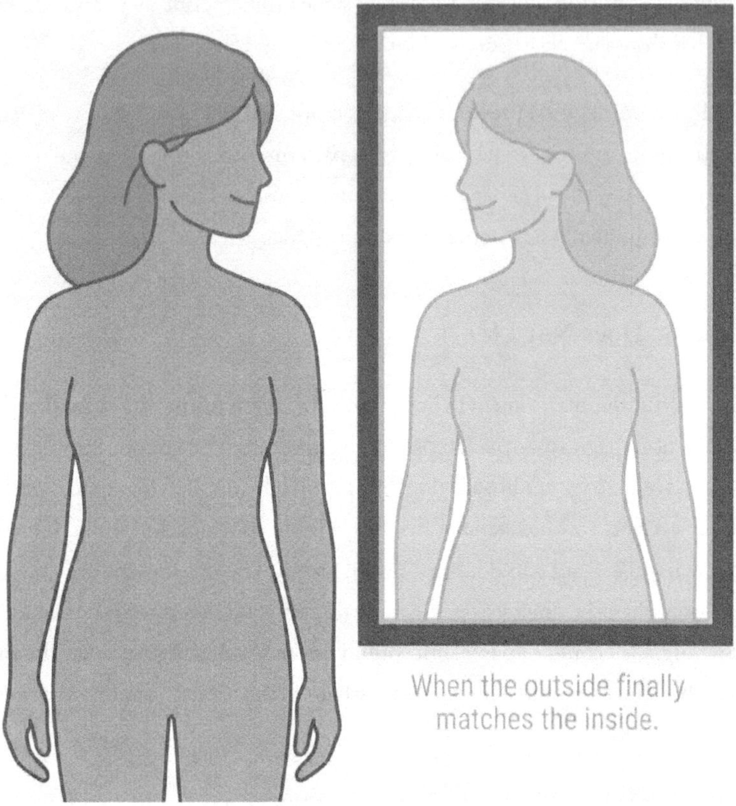

What Image Alignment Actually Feels Like

When alignment is present, I stop scanning myself like a problem to solve. The pieces—the skin, the hair, the energy, how I carry myself—stop being separate items on a mental checklist and become a seamless expression of who I am. I walk into rooms with presence rather than performance.

The confidence that comes from this is the quiet kind. Nothing to prove, no one to compete with, no trend to keep up with. It's the confidence of a woman who has earned her wisdom and genuinely likes who she sees. That kind of confidence is magnetic in a way no product can manufacture.

When alignment is off, I feel it before I can name it. It starts like a sliver—tiny, persistent, just below the surface. Eventually I can identify what needs attention. The goal of this chapter is to close that gap between how I feel inside and what I see outside. The heavy lifting is already done. Now I give the outside a chance to catch up.

The High-Maintenance / Low-Maintenance Approach

Full disclosure: I am an extremely low-maintenance person. This is ironic given my work in cosmetic medicine, but I have made my peace with it. My days are full, I'm always in a rush, and by the end I'm too tired for anything complicated.

I deeply admire women who can apply a full face of beautifully blended makeup in the morning and then follow it up with a twelve-step skincare routine at night.

I cannot. I am bare skin to the world approximately 95% of the time, and I've built a skincare approach that works for someone exactly like me. The interventions I choose are targeted and high-impact. The daily routine is minimal but non-negotiable.

Here's the honest secret: professional treatments can sometimes accomplish in one session what months of daily products can't—which keeps my morning routine blessedly short. More on those shortly.

My Non-Negotiable 1: Daily Sunscreen *(for discussion with your care provider)*

Not seasonal. Not optional on cloudy days. Not something you can "make up for later." A large share of visible facial aging is driven by cumulative sun exposure over time. Daily broad-spectrum sunscreen is one of the highest-return skincare investments at any price point.

For most people, a broad-spectrum SPF 30 or higher is a good baseline. Many prefer mineral formulas (often zinc oxide and/or titanium dioxide), especially if they're sensitive to certain chemical filters. The best sunscreen is the one I'll actually use—so the goal is to find one I genuinely like. If you do nothing else from this chapter, this one habit changes the trajectory of your skin for life.

My Non-Negotiable 2: Vitamin C *(for discussion with your care provider)*

Applied in the morning before sunscreen, vitamin C can help support brighter tone over time and can help the skin handle daily environmental stress. Think of it as the morning amplifier: sunscreen protects, vitamin C supports repair.

A note on tolerance: vitamin C can cause tingling, redness, or irritation—especially at higher strengths or on sensitive skin. Start low and build slowly. If you have reactive skin (or conditions like rosacea), please check with your clinician/dermatology provider before starting it.

My Non-Negotiable 3: Retinoids *(for discussion with your care provider)*

Retinoids (vitamin A–based ingredients) have some of the strongest evidence we have for improving texture, tone, and visible signs of aging over time.

Used in the evening, they can support healthier skin turnover and collagen signaling. Prescription tretinoin is often the most effective option; over-the-counter retinol is a gentler starting point. Of these 3 items, retinoids are most likely to cause irritation or intolerance. Begin slowly, under the guidance of your care provider—two to three nights per week—and build from there. Some initial dryness can happen. Consistency is the strategy, not suffering. Important: retinoids can be irritating and are not right for everyone. They're also not safe during pregnancy.

This is one product category where professional guidance genuinely matters—so please don't start one without discussing it with your care provider.

The Toothbrush Rule

Here is the real secret for staying consistent when I'm busy and tired: I do it while brushing my teeth. Cleanser while the toothbrush runs. Vitamin C serum while I rinse. Sunscreen while I look for my keys. Two minutes, zero extra time. Attaching a new habit to an existing one is one of the simplest ways to make it stick. It works.

A Brief Word on What to Avoid

If you have worked hard on your hormonal health, you do not want your skincare routine to accidentally make life harder. Some ingredients are common irritation triggers (especially added fragrance). Some people prefer to avoid certain preservatives or chemical UV filters that have raised questions in hormone-health circles.

You do not need a chemistry degree to make this practical: choosing fragrance-free when possible and sticking with a sunscreen you tolerate well covers a lot of ground. The workbook for this chapter includes a brand-neutral guide to reading skincare labels and sourcing quality products wherever you are in the world.

When the Daily Foundation Isn't Enough

Let's start with something nobody says out loud, but almost everyone feels the first time they consider walking into a clinic for an aesthetic treatment: *Is this going too far?*

For most women, the answer is no. But the fact that the question exists at all tells you something important about how we've been taught to think about self-care—and about ourselves.

Here is the reframe that changes everything: getting a professional aesthetic treatment is not categorically different from getting your hair colored, your nails done, or your lashes extended. Nobody agonizes over whether highlights make them shallow. Nobody feels they need to justify a good haircut. These are simply the ordinary, unremarkable ways that women who look after themselves look after themselves.

A laser appointment or a neuromodulator treatment belongs on exactly the same shelf. It is maintenance. It is the natural next step for a woman who has already done the hard internal work and is ready to let the outside fully reflect it, if and when it fits into her philosophy. The daily foundation we just discussed is the non-negotiable baseline. The professional layer is the amplifier—the option that does what no tube, serum, or home routine can do on its own. Not to change you. To restore you.

I want to tell you what I see when a woman comes in for her first appointment.

Laura is 47. She runs her own business—the kind where she's the brand, the operator, and the person who answers every email. Still, Laura still walks in a little unsure of whether she's allowed to be here.

There's a subtle hesitation in the way she settles into the chair.
A quiet apology woven into her first few sentences-like she needs to justify why she booked the appointment at all.

Underneath that, something deeper.

A flicker of guilt.
About spending money on herself.
On something that doesn't neatly fall into the category of "necessary."

Not groceries. Not school fees. Not something for everyone else.

Just... her.

There is a quiet worry about the slippery slope: *If I do this once, where does it end?* Underneath all of it, almost always, is the fear of coming out looking like someone else. Of losing the face that is recognizably, unmistakably hers.

I understand every one of those feelings. I do not have a smooth one-liner to dissolve them. What I do is normalize being there. I remind her that she has value too. That wanting to feel like what she sees in the mirror matches how she feels, is not a character flaw.

She is not here to be transformed—she is here to be restored.

What happens next is the part conventional medicine does not have a billing code for.

Sometimes the treatment is almost beside the point. What she really came for was a bit of time in a room where nobody needs anything from her, with someone who is genuinely glad she showed up. I have learned not to underestimate how much that matters. I am not just a provider. I am a witness. Sometimes that is the most important thing I can offer.

By the second appointment, she is usually smiling before she sits down. The apprehension is gone. She knows what to expect, she knows how she felt afterward, and she is ready. That shift—from hesitant to at home—is one of my favorite things to watch.

I Operate Without Operating

My clinical philosophy fits in four words: I operate without operating.

What that means in practice is that I work entirely within the non-surgical space—and I am honest about where that space ends. Non-surgical treatments are genuinely remarkable. They have changed what is possible for women who want to look refreshed, rested, and more like themselves with minimal downtime, surgery, or dramatic alteration. But they have limits.

Plastic surgeons still exist for very good reasons, and a provider who pretends otherwise—who promises surgical results from a needle or a device, who pushes treatments that are outside their scope because they do not want to refer you elsewhere—is not a provider you can trust.

The goal of everything I do is congruence. Not change. Most women who come to see me are not looking to look different. They are looking to look like themselves again—to reverse some unwanted change, to restore something that time or illness or stress quietly took.

The question I am always working from is: does this bring her closer to herself, or does it move her away? If the answer is the latter, I refer. Always. A good outcome means she leaves looking healthy, refreshed, and recognizably her—not done, not altered, not like a procedure happened. Just like herself on a very good day.

A red flag in any aesthetic consultation: a provider who recommends more than you asked for, pressures you toward same-day decisions, or makes you feel that your concerns are too minor or too significant for honest conversation. Trust your instincts. If something feels wrong, it probably is. You are always allowed to leave, think it over, and seek a second opinion. No legitimate provider will penalize you for taking time.

The Three Categories Worth Knowing

Rather than overwhelm you with a procedure catalogue—which would fill a book of its own—I want to give you a clear mental map of the three broad categories of non-surgical aesthetic treatment. This is enough to walk into any consultation anywhere in the world feeling oriented. The workbook for this chapter goes deeper on each one.

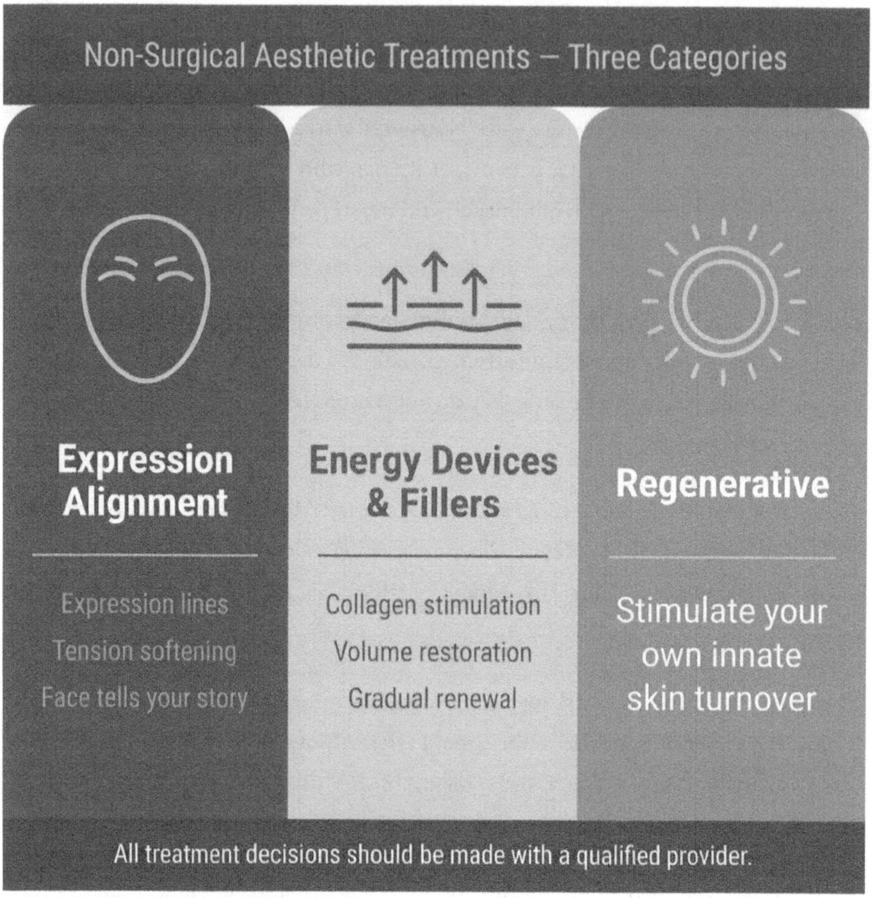

Category 1: Prevention and Expression Alignment

Neuromodulators—examples commonly known by brand names such as Botox or Xeomin, though availability varies by region—work by temporarily relaxing specific facial muscles that create expression lines.

Used well, they do not freeze the face or erase personality. They soften the lines that have formed from years of repeated movement and, more importantly, they can realign the outward expression with the inner one.

Here is a clinical example that captures why I love this treatment: some people spend years squinting and frowning while concentrating—perhaps they need glasses, perhaps it is just habit—and over time they develop deep lines between their brows that give the permanent outward appearance of being stern, unapproachable, or angry. They may be some of the warmest, most open-hearted people imaginable. But their face is telling a different story. A small amount of neuromodulator in exactly the right place closes that gap between who they are and what the world sees first. That is not vanity. That is communication.

On a personal note: I have used neuromodulators for years. What I did not expect was the added benefit of significantly reduced headaches—a well-documented secondary effect that I now consider as valuable as the cosmetic result.

Category 2: Energy Devices and Fillers

This category includes energy-based devices—lasers, light treatments, radiofrequency, and focused ultrasound—that work at various depths in the skin to stimulate the body's own collagen production, address pigmentation and texture, and provide gradual, natural-looking improvement over time.

My particular favorites are laser treatments for pigmentation and collagen stimulation, and focused ultrasound for deeper lifting and tightening. Focused ultrasound works gradually—results develop over several months as new collagen forms—and because the change is slow and incremental, it never distorts. You just look progressively more like yourself at your best.

For volume, fillers used conservatively restore what has been lost—in the cheeks, the temples, around the mouth—bringing back the facial proportions of a younger version of the same face. The operative word is conservatively. Overfilling is one of the most common and most avoidable aesthetic mistakes. Less is almost always more. The goal is restoration, not reconstruction.

Category 3: Your Body's Own Healing Power

The third category works by harnessing the body's own regenerative processes—using your own biology to stimulate repair, renewal, and collagen production from within.

This includes microneedling, platelet-rich plasma and platelet-rich fibrin treatments, some specialized fillers that stimulate collagen (biomodulation is the term used), polynucleotides, exosomes, and at the cutting edge— custom secretome treatments derived from your own banked stem cells. Stem cell banking is available now and allows you to preserve younger, more potent cells for use in increasingly sophisticated regenerative treatments as they continue to develop. It is simultaneously an aesthetic investment and a longevity investment.

Not Done. No Longer Sick – My Journey

After the cancer, after the tamoxifen, after the metabolic work that brought my body back—there was a new problem. My body looked healthy. My face looked like I had been sick.

The weight loss I had worked toward had taken facial volume with it, and what remained told a story I was finished living. I had done everything else. I had rebuilt from the inside out. Yet the mirror was still not reflecting the woman I had become.

So I did it. Filler to restore the volume that illness and weight loss had taken. Laser resurfacing for the skin quality that stress and cortisol and tamoxifen had eroded. A small amount of neuromodulator for the exhaustion lines that had taken up permanent residence. Not because I had a plan. Because I was frustrated and I knew what I needed and I was not willing to wait.

The result was subtle. That was the whole point. What I saw in the mirror afterward was not a procedure. It was not a transformation. It was a woman who looked healthy. Rested. Like herself—the self that had existed before the diagnosis, but with something extra. Something earned. I did not look younger. I looked well. I looked like I meant to still be here.

Not done. No longer sick. That was the moment. Everything on the inside had already changed. That afternoon in my own clinic, the outside finally caught up.

The Woman Who Closes the Tab

I want to speak directly to the woman who has been googling this at midnight and closing the tab before anyone sees. I know you are reading this book. I know you have done some of the work in the earlier chapters, maybe all of it. I know you have quietly wanted this for longer than you would admit. I know that what stops you is not the cost or the time or even the fear of the needle.

What stops you is the belief, absorbed so gradually you cannot remember when it started, that you are not quite deserving of it. That the money should go somewhere more important. That wanting to look good is indulgent in a way that wanting to feel good is not. That there are others whose needs come first—always, somehow, still.

This is not about cosmetic procedures. This is about anything that would bring you pleasure, joy, or care. It is the same pattern that keeps you from the doctor for years, from the gym for months, from the good night's sleep you kept promising yourself. The procedure is almost incidental.

The real question is whether you believe you are worth an hour of genuine attention.

My honest suggestion is not to book an appointment. It is to start somewhere quieter and more fundamental. To look at yourself—really look—and try to find the parts of yourself that are worthy of love and kindness. To begin speaking to yourself the way you would speak to a friend in the same position. To find your beginning, wherever it is, and take one small step from there.

The treatments will still be here when you are ready. When you arrive, it will not be because you finally caved to something superficial. It will be because you finally decided you are worth caring for. That is a completely different thing.

What Becomes Possible

When the inside-out work is in motion and the daily practice is in place, something shifts beyond the mirror. You walk into rooms differently—not louder, just more present. The quiet confidence of a woman with nothing to prove takes up space in the best possible way. You feel attractive again—not despite your age, but because of everything it represents. The wisdom. The perspective. The clarity about what matters.

Getting dressed becomes self-expression rather than negotiation.

Those bright, clear eyes? That is not the product of any serum. That is the outward expression of a woman who is sleeping well, living with purpose, and genuinely thriving from the inside out. No topical product can manufacture that. But the work you've done in this book already can.

Your Action for Today

One thing. Not a routine overhaul. Not a new regime starting Monday.

Find a sunscreen you actually like. Not the one from last summer at the back of the cabinet. Not the one that leaves a white cast or smells like a swimming pool. A good one—broad-spectrum, SPF 30 or higher—that you would genuinely reach for every morning without sighing. This one habit, done consistently, will do more for your skin over the next decade than almost anything else you can choose today.

Every morning when you put it on—even on a grey Tuesday when the hair is doing what it does and nothing feels particularly aligned—you are making a quiet declaration: *I am worth the two minutes. The sand in the hourglass is precious. I intend to make it count.*

Damn girl. You got this.

Your Chapter 10 Workbook Resources

The companion workbook turns this chapter into action. Scan the QR code below—or go to www.hotflashtohotdamnbook.com/workbook — to access the **Image Alignment Guide:** two practical resources in one—the Evidence-Based Skincare Guide and the Non-Surgical Treatment Overview, with questions to bring to any provider.

Chapter Eleven

The Cost of Waiting

What your future self needs you to understand

You have made it to Chapter 11. That means some part of you recognized yourself in these pages. It means you are not indifferent.

I have to say this, because I care too much not to: reading is not the same as beginning. Information is powerful-until it quietly becomes your favorite form of procrastination.

This chapter is not about pressure. It is not about urgency in the commercial sense-no countdown clock, no limited offer, no manufactured scarcity.

What it is about is something more fundamental and more honest than any of that: the biology of time. Because your body does not pause while you think it over. The slope of change does not wait for a convenient moment to become inconvenient. The distance between where you are and where you want to be can grow quietly, without announcement, with every month that passes.

That is not a threat. It is just the truth. You deserve the truth.

Why She Is Still Waiting

Let me be clear about something before we go any further: if you have been in research mode-reading, listening, learning, collecting information without yet acting on it-you are not failing. You are not weak or undisciplined or uncommitted. You are navigating a genuinely complicated landscape, and you have been doing it largely without adequate support.

The reasons women wait are real and varied. Some are overwhelmed by the volume of information and aren't sure where to begin-or in what sequence. Some have tried to raise these concerns with their doctors and been dismissed, rushed, or told their symptoms were "normal for their age." That response is common. It is also deeply unhelpful.

Some are afraid of change in the general sense-the quiet resistance that comes with stepping into unfamiliar territory. Some—many, in fact-are still carrying fear that was seeded by one study published in the early 2000s. The Women's Health Initiative (WHI) changed the conversation about hormone therapy almost overnight. The headlines were loud, fast, and scary. The follow-up nuance was... not. (That's not a criticism-it's just how media works. Corrections rarely trend.)

What's worth understanding now is that WHI studied specific hormone formulations and a population that, on average, was older and further from the menopausal transition than many of the women seeking symptom relief today. Important data-but not always a perfect match for the woman who hasn't slept in a year and is wondering if she's losing her mind.

Over the past two decades, the clinical conversation has evolved. Current menopause care is much more likely to focus on individualized risk assessment, shared decision-making, and the idea that age, time since menopause, dose, and route of delivery all matter. For many healthy, symptomatic women-especially earlier in the transition-hormone therapy can be a reasonable option.

For others, it isn't. The point isn't that hormones are "for everyone." The point is that the decision deserves an updated, individualized conversation-not one based on a headline you absorbed in a different decade of your life. So if you've been cautious because of what you heard years ago, that doesn't make you wrong. It makes you human.

But you're also allowed to revisit the conversation with current information and a clinician who will weigh what's true for you. If you have been afraid of hormone therapy based on what you heard or read years ago, you are not wrong to have been cautious. You were responding to the information available to you.

But the information has changed. You are allowed to change with it.

The Slope of the Curve

What we're dealing with is a trajectory. Not a cliff edge, not a sudden catastrophe-a slope. What treatment and well-sequenced care can do is change the angle of that slope.

When the hormonal transition goes unaddressed, the losses-in bone density, muscle mass, cardiovascular protection, cognitive sharpness, metabolic function, mood stability, and sleep quality-tend to happen faster than they need to.

When we intervene thoughtfully, we flatten the curve. We reduce the rate of loss. We protect what's already there. Here's the part most women are quietly asking (even if they don't say it out loud): does it really matter when I start? The compassionate, honest answer is yes-it matters. Not because you've failed if you haven't started yet, and not because you need to panic. It matters because earlier tends to protect more. It also matters to hear the second half of that sentence, because this is where women get stuck: later still helps-often meaningfully.

Starting now can still improve sleep, steadiness, quality of life, and long-term health markers. What changes with earlier support is not whether you can benefit-it's how much you're able to protect.

Another honest truth: some things take longer to rebuild than they would have taken to protect. That isn't a scare tactic. It's just how physiology works. It's easier to preserve muscle than to rebuild it after years of disrupted sleep and declining hormones. It's easier to protect bone than to try to catch up after a bigger loss. It's easier to support cognition when you're sleeping well than when you've been white-knuckling 3 a.m. for two years. So no-this isn't "now or never." It's "now protects more." You deserve to make that decision with clarity, not fear.

The good news is real: it is almost never too late to change the slope. The curve can be flattened at almost any point. The question isn't whether you can improve. The question is simply: how much do you want to protect starting now?

The Five Windows: Where Timing Has the Most Leverage

The slope we have been discussing is not one uniform decline. It is made up of specific domains—each with its own timeline and its own window where support makes the biggest difference. These are not deadlines. They are not ultimatums. They are simply the biology of when intervention protects the most.

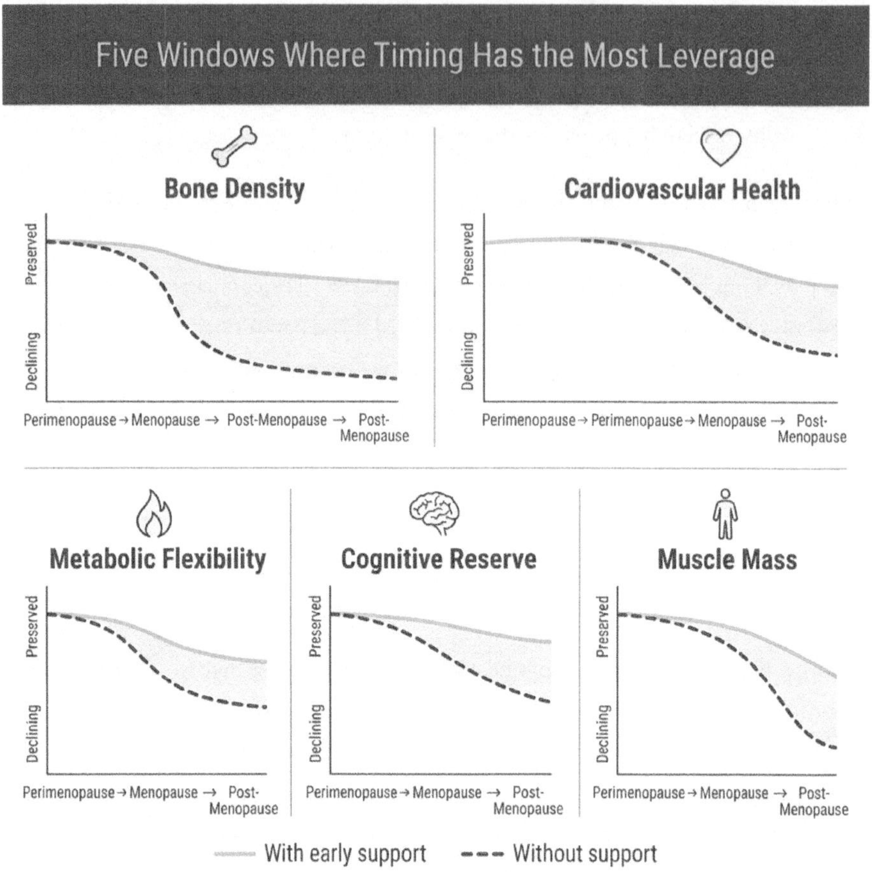

Bone Density. Bone loss accelerates significantly in the first five to seven years after menopause. This is the window where protective measures—weight-bearing exercise, adequate calcium and vitamin D, and when appropriate, hormonal support—have the most impact. Once significant bone loss has occurred, rebuilding is possible but slower and harder than preserving what was already there.

Cardiovascular Health. Research suggests that hormone therapy initiated within ten years of menopause onset, or before the age of sixty, may have the most favorable cardiovascular risk profile. This is sometimes called the "timing hypothesis." After that window, the risk-benefit calculation shifts. This does not mean hormones become dangerous later—it means the cardiovascular protective benefit is strongest when support begins early.

Metabolic Flexibility. Your body's ability to switch smoothly between burning carbohydrates and burning fat—metabolic flexibility—becomes less responsive over time, especially when compounded by poor sleep, chronic stress, and hormonal decline. Addressing these upstream conditions earlier in the transition preserves more metabolic adaptability. The longer these patterns entrench, the harder they are to shift.

Cognitive Reserve. Brain health is cumulative. Sleep quality, exercise, hormonal support, and stress management in midlife are among the strongest modifiable factors for long-term cognitive function. The evidence does not suggest that midlife decline is inevitable—it suggests that what you do now builds or depletes a reserve your brain will draw on for decades.

Muscle Mass. Sarcopenia—age-related muscle loss—accelerates after fifty. Strength training and adequate protein intake in midlife are the most effective countermeasures we have. Muscle is not just about aesthetics. It is metabolic currency: it regulates blood sugar, protects joints, supports bone density, and is one of the strongest predictors of quality of life in later decades. The earlier you start building and preserving it, the more you keep.

None of these are deadlines. All of them respond to intervention at almost any point. But the return on investment is highest when you start early—and you deserve to make that decision with the specifics in front of you, not just a vague sense that "earlier is better."

Natalie

Natalie came in on a Tuesday afternoon in November, referred by her GP with a note that said simply: perimenopausal symptoms, not coping well.

She was 55. A financial consultant. The kind of woman people describe as unflappable-because she usually is. She had a husband she loved, adult kids, and the quiet logistics of midlife: her mother in assisted living, a calendar that never seemed to get lighter, and a brain that was used to solving problems.

Inside, she had not slept through the night in two years. She was waking four and five times, drenched, heart pounding, lying in the dark at 3 a.m. with a mind that would not power down. She had started keeping a change of pajamas on the bedside table. Her husband had moved to the spare room-not out of unkindness, but because they were both exhausted and at least one of them needed to sleep.

At work, she started writing everything down. Not because she had ever been disorganized-she'd built a whole career on being sharp-but because words were slipping. Names. The thread of a sentence midway through a meeting. She started arriving early to presentations to run through notes again, terrified of the moment her mind would go blank in front of a room full of people who expected her certainty.

Then there was the part she didn't know how to explain without sounding dramatic: the morning joint aches. The weight gain that didn't make sense given how disciplined she was. The anxiety-unfamiliar and unsettling-like her body was quietly ringing an alarm that nobody else could hear. She had mentioned it to her previous doctor eighteen months earlier.

She'd been told her bloodwork was normal, this was a natural part of aging, and many women found it helpful to reduce stress. She left the appointment feeling quietly ashamed-like the appropriate response to what she was experiencing was better self-management.

She didn't go back. She read instead. Articles, books, podcasts, forums. She accumulated enough information to understand what might be happening-but no clear order of operations. Every answer introduced another variable. Every test suggestion raised new concerns. She didn't need more information. She needed a doorway. A map. When she finally sat down across from me that Tuesday, she said something I have heard in many different forms from many different women: "I think I waited too long. I think I've done damage I can't undo."

She hadn't waited too long. But she had waited longer than she needed to. The losses she was worried about-the sleep debt, the cognitive load, the stress on her marriage, the quiet erosion of confidence-those were real. Some would resolve quickly. Some would take longer to rebuild than they would have taken to protect. Within a few weeks of starting a plan that fit her physiology, she sent a message through the clinic portal. Four words: I slept last night. From there, the up-spiral began. Better sleep created bandwidth. Bandwidth created capacity. Capacity created strength. Somewhere in the middle of that, the anxiety often eased-not because life became perfect, but because she finally had a roadmap.

The Only Reframe That Matters

I could build a clinical case for early intervention. I could walk you through the compounding returns of the up-spiral we just watched Natalie begin. But none of that is the real answer to why now. She deserves it.

You deserve it. Not because you have earned it through sufficient suffering. Not because you have done enough research to justify the investment. Not because your symptoms have finally crossed some threshold of severity that makes seeking help acceptable. Simply because you are a human being, living one life, and that life deserves your full attention and your best care. You do not need to explain wanting to feel well. You do not need to justify seeking treatment for a physiological transition that is affecting your quality of life. You do not need permission from anyone-not your partner, not your mother, not the voice in your head that has been telling you for years that other people's needs come first. You are not on that list by accident. You belong on it. The overwhelm is real, but it does not get to make this decision for you.

The broken medical system is real, but it does not get to make this decision for you. The old fear about hormones is understandable, but it is based on information that has been substantially corrected, and it does not get to make this decision for you either.

You get to make this decision. You get to make it now.

What Happens When You Begin

For the woman who is close but not yet certain, here is what often happens when you begin-not perfectly, not all at once, just intentionally. The first shift is usually not dramatic. It's relief. You stop feeling like you're fighting a mystery with willpower and Google tabs. You get a plan. You get a next step. You get your nervous system out of "guessing mode."

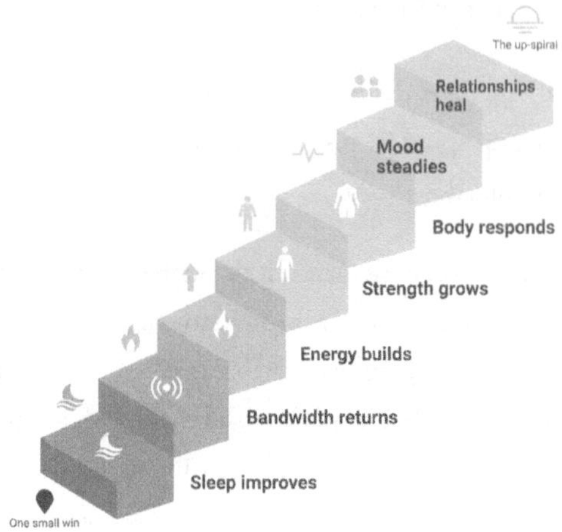

Each win makes the next one possible

Then the symptoms that have been running the show-hot flashes, disrupted sleep, mood swings, that edgy "why am I like this?" feeling-often start to soften. Not because you've suddenly become more disciplined, but because your physiology is finally being supported in the right order. Here's where it compounds: when sleep improves even a little, you get bandwidth.

With bandwidth, you can walk. When you walk, you get a bit of energy back. With energy, you can lift. When you lift, your body composition can shift. When your body changes, your mood changes.

When your mood changes, your relationships change. It's not magic. It's physiology. It's the up-spiral: one small win makes the next one possible. This is why starting matters. Not because you need to do everything. But because you deserve to feel the first win-the one that proves to your brain and body: Oh. This is actually doable. If systemic hormone therapy isn't right for you-because of your medical history, your risk factors, your preferences, or simply where you are in the decision-please hear me: you are not out of options.

Non-hormonal approaches can meaningfully support symptoms and quality of life, and the foundational levers still "count" in a big way: protecting sleep, building strength, stabilizing stress, and eating in a way that supports muscle and metabolism. If vaginal or urinary symptoms are part of your picture, local (non-systemic) therapies are often a separate conversation-one you can explore with your clinician based on your specific situation. The on-ramp might look different, but you can still begin-and beginning still changes the slope.

The One Thing

If I had thirty seconds with every woman who has ever picked up this book, worked up the courage to read it all the way through, and then talked herself out of acting on it during the drive home, I would say this: This is your only life. One time around. No do-overs. You cannot change your past, but your future is not written. You deserve the best life you can have. You are worthy of that. All of it-the health, the energy, the clarity, the confidence, the joy-is possible.

But it requires you to decide that you are worth beginning for. The slope is real. The window of maximum protection is real. But so is the capacity to flatten the curve at almost any point. So is the up-spiral. So is the woman who walks into her follow-up differently than she walked into her first appointment-not because she was "fixed," but because she remembered something important about herself. That woman is not a lucky exception. She is a predictable outcome of a woman who decided, on one ordinary day, that she was worth the phone call.

Your One Action

Not a program. Not a complete overhaul. Not a commitment to everything at once. One phone call. Call your primary care physician, your nurse practitioner, your GP, your gynecologist-whoever is the most accessible door into your healthcare.

You do not have to know exactly what you want yet. You do not have to arrive with a diagnosis or a treatment plan or a list of demands. You just have to show up and say: "I've been reading about perimenopause and menopause, and I think it's time for us to talk." That is the whole assignment. One call. One conversation you have been putting off that no longer needs to hold you.

You have the tools. You have the Three-Goal Rule from Chapter 7 and the Power Phrase Bank to help you advocate for yourself in that room. You have the framework from Chapter 8 to understand how the pieces connect. You have the workbooks. You have the knowledge. Use that. Walk in prepared, clear, and without apology. You have earned the right to be heard.

You Do Not Have to Walk It Alone

You have everything you need-the knowledge, the framework, the workbooks, the tools. But some paths are easier with company. If you find yourself at a crossroads-if you hit a wall with your provider, if the system pushes back, if you aren't sure which step comes next or how to sequence what you've learned-I would be genuinely honored to walk alongside you. Not because you need rescuing, but because this work is better when it is shared. You will find me through the QR code below. No pressure, no obligation, no urgency beyond the one that is already yours: the quiet knowledge that your future self is counting on the decision you make now.

Your Chapter 11 Workbook Resource

The companion workbook turns this chapter into action. Scan the QR code below—or go to www.hotflashtohotdamnbook.com/workbook — to access the **Cost of Waiting Inventory and Window of Leverage:** a guided reflection to help you identify what has been keeping you waiting and what your next right step actually is.

Chapter Twelve

The Phoenix

You were always going to rise.

Do you remember the woman who opened this book? She was frustrated. Worn down. Carrying a quiet grief she could not quite name, a gap between who she used to be and who she had become.

She had tried things that did not work, navigated a system that let her down, and wondered more than once whether the woman she used to be was simply gone.

But she had something else too. A flicker. A small, stubborn belief that things could be different. That somewhere there was an answer nobody had given her yet. That woman picked up this book. That decision—that single act of choosing to seek rather than accept—was the first step of everything that followed.

Look at where you are now. You have not just read twelve chapters. You have started something. The momentum is already moving, and here is what I need you to understand about momentum: it does not stop on its own. It builds.

Every step forward creates the conditions for the next one. Every piece of knowledge you have absorbed, every reflection that landed, every moment you recognized yourself in these pages—all of it is already working. You are already different from the woman who opened to page one. The momentum has started. You are unstoppable.

The Woman You Are Becoming

I want you to close your eyes for a moment and find her. Not the woman you were before the exhaustion set in—someone new. Someone forged from everything you have been through and everything you now know. She lives a congruent life. Not perfect—congruent. Her outside matches her inside. Her choices match her values. The time and energy she gives match what she has decided actually deserves them.

She has stopped spending herself on things and people that diminish her, and started investing in the ones that fill her. She values and honors her body. She nourishes it, moves it, rests it, tends to it—not out of discipline or punishment but out of genuine respect for the life it carries. She dresses it with care. She sees it with kindness. She no longer makes herself wait. Her relationships are deeper. Chosen deliberately. Built on mutual respect rather than obligation. She is more present in them—because she is more present in herself.

She knows the tools by name now. The CLEAR Framework, for the moments when she needs to protect her energy without burning the relationship. The Three-Goal Rule, for the appointments where she used to leave empty-handed. The Daily Cortisol Reset, for the days when the stress chemistry gets loud before she does. The Four-Layer Reset, for the times when her body stops cooperating and she needs to know which lever to pull first. These are not concepts. They are her operating system now. And unlike the coping strategies she used before — the ones built on willpower and performance and the quiet hope that nobody would notice — this one was built for the woman she actually is. It runs on precision. It runs on sequence. And it runs on the knowledge that she has never been the problem.

The energy she reclaimed through this work does not disappear into a void. It flows outward, into the people and moments that matter most, enriching everything it touches. She is fulfilled- not in a destination, as a daily reality. The sun is shining within her regardless of the weather outside. That woman is not a fantasy. She is you — already in motion, already on her way. Now, it is time to set down the last thing that has been slowing her down.

The Lie You Can Finally Set Down

You have been carrying something that was never yours to carry. The belief that your value lives in your service. That you are only as worthy as what you do for others, only as deserving as the care you provide, only as acceptable as your usefulness allows. It was handed to you so early and so thoroughly that you stopped questioning it.

It shaped everything—who you put first, what you allowed yourself to want, how long you waited before asking for help. That lie has had its last day. What is true—what has always been true, whether you felt it or not—is that you are inherently valuable. Not because of what you produce or who you care for. Simply because you exist. Your worth is not something you earn or maintain or prove. It is something you are. You were valuable before you did a single thing for anyone. You will be valuable long after the caregiving is done. That was never in question. It just took twelve chapters to finally let it land.

The Truth You Get to Live By

Your past does not control your future. Whatever the trajectory was before you opened this book—the decline, the slope, the accumulation of years of unaddressed hormonal change and chronic stress and self-neglect and a medical system that did not have answers—that trajectory has changed. The moment you chose to begin, the angle shifted. You do not have to undo everything that came before. You just have to hold the new direction.

This is your north star. When the system pushes back, return to it. When the old voice gets loud, return to it. When the guilt resurfaces and the list of everyone else's needs grows longer than the day, return to it. Your past does not control your future. The best of it is still unwritten. You are the one holding the pen.

Just One More Step

Here is what I want you to do when you close this book. Not a program. Not a complete overhaul. Not a commitment to everything at once. Just one more step—whatever the next step is from exactly where you are standing right now. If you have not yet made the call, make the call. Pick up the phone, reach whoever is the most accessible door into your care, and make the appointment. That is the whole step.

If you have made the call, prepare for the appointment. Sit with a piece of paper and write the real version—not the minimized, curated version designed not to be a burden, but the honest one. Where are you actually struggling? What do you most need someone to hear?

That is your preparation. That is your power.

If you have already done that, then your step is this: close your eyes and find the woman you are becoming. See her clearly. Feel what it feels like to be her. Carry that image into the appointment with you and let it give you what you need—the strength, the courage, the quiet authority of a woman who knows what she deserves and is done settling for less.

One step. Just one.

That is how it begins. No magic. No perfect moment.

Just a woman who decides, on one ordinary day, that she is worth the next step.

The Fire

I want to tell you something that has never fit inside a clinical framework.

I have been through my own fire. Cancer. Tamoxifen. Induced menopause. Relationships cut away because I could no longer afford the cost of them. A divorce. Years of self-doubt I did not even recognize until the fire burned them off.

I cannot put into words how painful it was. What I will tell you is what came through it.

Clarity. Strength I did not know I had. A life that is brighter, closer, and more real than anything before it—because I stopped wasting myself on things and people that did not deserve me. Work that fills me. Relationships deeper than anything I had before, precisely because they survived something that cost everything.

I would never wish that fire on anyone.

I would also not trade what it made me.

Here is what I know about the phoenix: once it burns, it cannot recreate what came before. What rises from the ashes is something completely new. That is not a loss—it is the point.

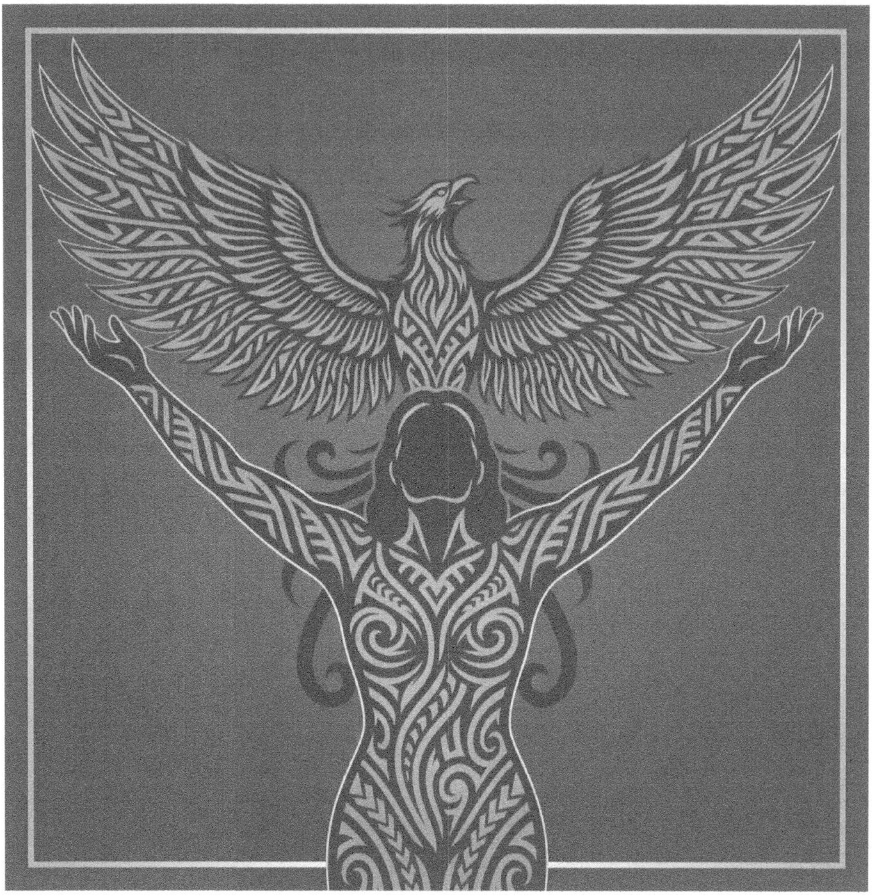

You cannot un-see what you now see. You cannot un-know your own worth.

The woman who closes this book is not the same woman who opened it, and there is no going back to who she was before. Not because she is leaving something behind, but because she is finally, fully, arriving somewhere.

I wish that for you. The clarity, the strength, the life that is brighter and closer and real. I believe, with everything I have, that it is already yours.

You just have to keep walking toward it.

Before You Close This Book

I want to ask one thing of you. Think of your very best friend in the whole world. She is the one you would go to the ends of the earth for. The one whose worth you have never once questioned, whose pain you feel as your own, who you would fight the whole broken system on behalf of without a second thought. You would never tell her she had to earn the right to feel well. You would never put her last. Now, understand that the woman I am describing is you.

Now give that to yourself. Stop waiting to earn the care you need. Stop making yourself prove that your symptoms are serious enough, your needs justified enough, your desire to feel well reasonable enough. You do not have to earn any of it. You never did. You have spent a lifetime being someone else's person. It is time—long past time—to be your own. Be your own best friend. Starting today.

You Are Not Walking Alone

You have everything you need. The knowledge, the framework, the workbooks, the tools—all of it is in your hands. Your local care team is your home base. This book was written to support that relationship, and most of what you need is available right where you are.

But if you need more—if the door does not open easily, if you want guidance before your appointment, or simply want company from someone who has walked this road—I am here.

Not as an obligation, just as an open door in whatever form fits where you are. For readers in parts of Canada, that can include working together directly within my medical practice. For readers anywhere in the world, it can include one-to-one coaching, self-paced courses, and the lab-based education program we built to help you understand your own biology

Where to start?

Path 1—Start With Your Labs: If you want to start by understanding your own hormones before your appointment, the lab-based education program pairs a hormone panel with a self-guided video series that teaches you the vocabulary — what each hormone does, what typical ranges look like, and what questions each value might prompt. With that understanding in hand, you can bring your results back to your own physician, or if you are in Canada, you can bring them into my medical practice for clinical follow-up. This is right for you if you want to understand what is actually happening in your body before you commit to a program—you need data before you can trust a direction.

Path 2—The Precision Hormone Course: This is right for you if you are self-directed, you have done the reading, and you want to go deeper at your own pace and on your own schedule. If you want to go deeper into everything this book covers, my full course—with video modules and a private support community—is available to you.

Path 3—Work With Me Directly: This is right for you if you are done figuring this out alone and you want ongoing support as you navigate your care.

For readers anywhere in the world, that support looks like one-to-one coaching. We work through your results together, prepare you for your appointments, help you build a self-advocacy strategy, and give you a framework to keep making sense of what your body is telling you. Coaching is educational and supportive. It does not replace the diagnosis, interpretation, or treatment that your own physician provides.

For readers in Canada, there is a second door. You can also come directly into my medical practice, where we can work together as physician and patient within the full scope of clinical care.

Two different kinds of support. Both real. Both designed to meet you where you are.

Or you can simply follow along. A little moral support in the background costs nothing and keeps our connection alive.

Whatever level of support fits your life right now—it exists, it is available, and it comes from the same place this book came from: a genuine wish to see you well.

Your Chapter 12 Workbook Resource

The companion workbook turns this chapter into action. Scan the QR code below—or go to www.hotflashtohotdamnbook.com/workbook — to access the **Phoenix Rising Plan**: your forward-looking commitment tool, with space to name where you are, where you're going, and how you intend to get there.

The woman who picked up this book on one ordinary day—tired, frustrated, quietly certain that something was wrong that nobody had been able to explain—she did not come this far to stop here. She came this far because some part of her always knew that better was possible. That part was right. It always was. The door is open. The path is yours. I will be right there with you when you walk through it. Now go.

About the Author

Amber Bocknek, MD spent years on the right side of the exam table — the one with the credentials and the prescription pad — before she ended up on the wrong side of it. Graves' disease she diagnosed as too much Tim Hortons. Breast cancer she found on a fax she read before the paper cleared the tray. Breast-cancer-treatment-induced menopause that took her hormones overnight and gave her 45 pounds she didn't ask for. A medical system she had trained in, trusted, and built her career within — one that had not yet integrated the answers she needed most.

So she went looking. Functional medicine. Hormonal sequencing. The research on bioidentical hormone replacement therapy that was not yet part of her training. She rebuilt her clinical framework from the ground up — and, piece by piece, rebuilt herself into the kind of physician who had been the patient and was done watching other women get lost in the same gaps the system left her in.

She founded Thrive! MedAesthetics + Wellness Ltd. in Aurora, Ontario, where she practices whole-woman care that looks at every layer simultaneously and takes the time to build a plan around each woman, not around a protocol. She sees patients in Canada, coaches clients globally through the Precision Hormone Program, and hosts *Longevanity*, a podcast on healthspan and youthfulness.

When she is not in the clinic, she is near water, playing harp (acoustic and electric, because one was not enough), kite-surfing with more enthusiasm than skill, or negotiating with one of the four cats who share her home and answer to no one. Her husband Jory is a veterinarian — he handles the patients with four legs; she handles the ones with two. It works beautifully, except possibly for the cats.

Amber Bocknek, MD, CCFP, practising in hormone health and longevity, ABAARM, FAAMM, MSCP, is a board-certified family physician and Menopause Society Certified Practitioner. *HOT Flash to HOT DAMN!* is her first book.

Review Request

One Last Thing

If this book found you at the right moment, pass it to the next woman who needs it. Your recommendation to a friend, sister, or colleague is how this work reaches the people it was written for.

And if a short Amazon review is easier than a conversation, that is welcome too—please review the book as you would any other book you have read, simply letting future readers know whether it was a useful resource.

Leave a book review: www.hotflashtohotdamnbook.com/review

From the bottom of my heart: thank you for being here.

Let's Connect & Continue the Journey

Working With Amber Bocknek, MD

You just finished a book that gave language to what your body has been telling you. The research. The physiology. The system that has let too many women fall through the cracks. The woman you have been underneath all of it—the one who was never broken, just unsupported.

You felt something while you read it. Maybe recognition. Maybe relief. Maybe anger at how long you went without this information. Maybe, for the first time in a long time, hope.

That feeling is not the finish line. It is the starting gun.

Your most important next step

Call your primary care provider. This week. Not when you feel ready. Not after you have done more research. Not once things slow down. Now.

Bring this book. Bring your symptom list. Bring the questions from Chapter 7. Bring the lab prep sheets from the workbook. You have everything you need to walk into that appointment differently than you have walked into every appointment before—informed, prepared, and unwilling to leave without a plan.

That conversation is where your journey moves from reading to real. That is the single most important thing you can do this week.

If that door does not open

Here is what I have learned working with women across every stage of this journey: the women who get the best outcomes are not the ones who know the most. They are the ones who feel supported enough to keep going when it gets hard.

Sometimes your primary care provider is exactly the right partner for that. Sometimes, despite your best efforts and the most prepared appointment of your life, you leave feeling unheard. If that happens, it is not the end of the road. It is simply a sign that you need a different door.

The Precision Hormone Program was built for that moment.

It is the coaching framework that applies the principles of this book to your life—a structured, whole-woman approach that helps you understand your own physiology, prepare for productive conversations with your physician, and build a self-advocacy plan you can actually use. Coaching is educational and supportive. It is not a replacement for clinical diagnosis, interpretation, or treatment, which belongs in the physician–patient relationship you have with your own provider. For readers in Canada, clinical care is also available inside my medical practice, where we can work together as physician and patient within the full scope of that relationship.

The door is open regardless of where you live.

What the Precision Hormone Program addresses

This program was built for a specific landscape. For women whose symptoms have been dismissed or normalized despite years of "your labs look fine." For women who have moved, lost their family doctor, or cannot find a provider willing to engage seriously with hormonal health. For women who have done the reading, done the guessing, done the trying—and still cannot get a clear picture of what is happening inside their own bodies.

The coaching framework examines four layers: your symptom pattern, your lab picture, your lifestyle context, and the gap between what you are experiencing and what the current system has been able to offer you. It gives you the vocabulary, the questions, and the self-advocacy tools to walk into any medical appointment as a more informed participant in your own care. For readers in Canada who need clinical follow-through, that can also happen inside my medical practice.

The framework does not promise outcomes. No program can. What it offers is a structured, whole-woman approach built on the same principles as the book, applied with the benefit of one-to-one support.

The door is open

You do not have to have it all figured out before you visit the page. The page is designed to help you figure it out.

Come as you are. Come with questions. Come with your lab results or come empty-handed. The woman who walks through that door is the same woman who picked up this book—the one who decided, on one ordinary day, that she was worth beginning for.

That decision brought you here. The next one takes you forward. I will see you on the other side.

Amber Bocknek, MD, CCFP, practising in hormone health and longevity. MSCP, A4M Fellow, Wellness Coach Certified by Mayo Clinic, CWC.

Your next step is simple. Go to www.hotflashtohotdamnbook.com/workbook and download the free companion workbook. It turns every chapter into action and it is waiting for you right now.

Once you have worked through the workbook, your results will tell you exactly which of the three paths forward is the right one for you—and everything you need to take that step is waiting at www.precisionlongevity.life/precision-hormone-profile

We can also stay in touch via socials and the web:

- **Website:** www.thriveaurora.com (clinical site) and www.precisionlongevity.life (coaching site)
- **Podcast:** Longevanity | YouTube and all major podcast platforms

- **Instagram:** @dramberbocknekmd | @thrive_aurora | @myprecisionlongevity
- **Facebook:** Amber Bocknek, MD | Thrive Aurora **LinkedIn:** Amber Bocknek, MD
- **Workbook:** https://hotflashtohotdamnbook.com/workbook

Recommended Reading and References

For the Reader Who Wants to Go Deeper

This book was written to give you a framework—a way of understanding what is happening in your body and why, and a map for moving through it with more clarity than the system typically offers. What it could not do is go everywhere. There is a large and growing body of excellent clinical and research literature on perimenopause, menopause, hormone health, and the full-body systems covered in these chapters.

What follows is a curated list of the resources I return to, assign to patients, and recommend without reservation. They are organized by category so you can find what is most relevant to where you are in your own journey.

Books

Hormones and Menopause—Clinical Foundation

The Menopause Brain—Lisa Mosconi, PhD (2024)

- Groundbreaking neuroscience on how menopause is a brain event as much as a hormonal one. Dr. Mosconi directs the Women's Brain Initiative at Weill Cornell and her research on estrogen, cognitive health, and Alzheimer's risk prevention is important work in this space right now. Required reading if you are concerned about brain fog, memory, or long-term cognitive protection.

Estrogen Matters—Avrum Bluming, MD and Carol Tavris, PhD (revised 2024)

- The definitive dissection of the Women's Health Initiative and the misinformation that followed it. A medical oncologist and a social psychologist together make the clearest evidence-based case for hormone therapy I have encountered in print. If you or your provider have concerns about HRT and breast cancer risk, start here.

The New Menopause—Mary Claire Haver, MD (2024)

- A comprehensive, accessible, and clinically rigorous guide to every dimension of menopause from a board-certified OB/GYN and Certified Menopause Provider. Covers bone health, cardiovascular risk, genitourinary syndrome, hormone therapy options, and self-advocacy. A strong companion to this book for the reader who wants more clinical detail.

The Menopause Manifesto—Jen Gunter, MD (2021)

- A frank, evidence-based, and unapologetically feminist deconstruction of menopause medicine—what we know, what has been withheld, and why. Dr. Gunter is a gynecologist and a skilled medical communicator. Strong on the history of how menopause became a neglected clinical area and what it will take to change that.

The Definitive Guide to the Perimenopause and Menopause—Louise Newson, MD (revised 2024)

- Dr. Newson is the UK's leading menopause specialist and the founder of Newson Health. This comprehensive guide covers physical, psychological, relational, and professional dimensions of the transition. Particularly useful on HRT dosing, testosterone, and the neurodivergent brain in menopause—an underserved area she has brought important research to.

Thyroid, Cortisol, and the HPA Axis

Why Do I Still Have Thyroid Symptoms When My Lab Tests Are Normal?—Datis Kharrazian, DHSc, DC, MS (2010)

- The book I recommend most often to women who have been told their thyroid is normal and do not believe it. Kharrazian makes the clinical case for why a standard TSH test misses the majority of thyroid dysfunction, and what a complete picture actually looks like. Dense but accessible, and worth every page.

Hormone Intelligence—Aviva Romm, MD (2021)

- A thorough integrative medicine guide to the full hormonal ecosystem—cortisol, thyroid, estrogen, progesterone, insulin—and how they interact across a woman's lifespan. Dr. Romm is a physician and herbalist whose approach bridges functional and conventional medicine in a way that is clinically grounded and practically useful.

Longevity, Healthspan, and Precision Medicine

The XX Brain—Lisa Mosconi, PhD (2020)

- Dr. Mosconi's earlier work on the female brain and Alzheimer's prevention. Focuses on nutrition, lifestyle, and the specific vulnerabilities of the female brain across the lifespan. A strong companion to The Menopause Brain for women who want to understand the cognitive dimension of their hormonal health in depth.

Clinical Organizations and Position Statements

These are the primary clinical bodies whose evidence-based position statements inform hormone therapy practice. Their websites offer patient-facing resources, provider directories, and the most current consensus guidelines.

The Menopause Society (formerly NAMS)

Website: menopause.org

- North America's leading nonprofit in menopause medicine. Their 2022 Hormone Therapy Position Statement and 2023 Nonhormone Therapy Position Statement are the clinical gold standard on which evidence-based prescribing is based. The site includes the MenoNote patient handout series—clear, well-sourced summaries on specific topics including the decision about hormone therapy, vaginal health, bone health, and more. If you want to bring something to a provider appointment, start here.

The Institute for Functional Medicine (IFM)

Website: ifm.org

Key resource: ifm.org/articles/menopause-hormone-therapy

- The leading training body for functional medicine physicians. Their articles and clinical tools on hormone therapy, the HPATG axis (hypothalamic-pituitary-adrenal-thyroid-gonadal), thyroid dysfunction beyond TSH, and the interconnected nature of hormonal systems are some of the most clinically practical resources available outside of peer-reviewed journals. The IFM blog covers cortisol, thyroid, estrogen metabolism, gut health and hormones, and precision diagnostics—exactly the upstream work covered in this book.

The American Academy of Anti-Aging Medicine (A4M)

Blog: blog.a4m.com

- A4M brings together the leading practitioners in hormonal optimization, longevity medicine, and precision health. Their blog covers hormone therapy, metabolic health, peptide therapy, healthspan optimization, and the evolving evidence base for women's health at midlife—including timely updates on FDA regulatory changes to HRT. For the reader who wants to track the frontier of what is changing in this field, the A4M blog is one of the best ongoing resources available.

The Society of Obstetricians and Gynaecologists of Canada (SOGC)

Website: sogc.org

- For Canadian readers: the SOGC publishes clinical practice guidelines on menopause management that are specific to the Canadian healthcare context. Their menopause committee guidelines align closely with NAMS and provide a useful framework for conversations with Canadian providers about what is available and covered in your province.

Key Clinical Studies and Position Papers

These are the landmark studies and consensus documents that the clinical guidance in this book is built on. You do not need to read them in full—but knowing they exist, and that the recommendations in these pages are grounded in peer-reviewed evidence, matters.

- *The 2022 Hormone Therapy Position Statement of The North American Menopause Society.* Menopause, 2022. pubmed.ncbi.nlm.nih.gov/35797481

• *The 2023 Nonhormone Therapy Position Statement of The North American Menopause Society.* Menopause, 2023. pubmed.ncbi.nlm.nih.gov/37252752

• *Crandall CJ, Mehta JM, Manson JE. Management of menopausal symptoms: a review.* JAMA, 2023; 329(5):405-420. The current state-of-the-art clinical summary on treating vasomotor symptoms and the full range of menopause management options.

• *Mosconi L et al. Menopause impacts human brain structure, connectivity, energy metabolism, and amyloid-beta deposition.* Scientific Reports, 2021. The landmark neuroimaging study demonstrating that menopause produces measurable changes in the female brain—not just in the ovaries.

• *IFM Menopause Hormone Therapy: Weighing Benefits and Risks.* Institute for Functional Medicine. ifm.org/articles/menopause-hormone-therapy

Websites and Ongoing Resources

Let's Talk Menopause

letstalkmenopause.org

• A nonprofit organization producing evidence-based patient education, podcast content featuring leading researchers, and advocacy for better menopause care. One of the highest-quality consumer-facing resources in this space.

Newson Health—Balance App and Resource Library

drlouisenewson.co.uk

• Dr. Louise Newson's clinic and patient platform, including the Balance app for symptom tracking. The resource library covers a wide range of topics from HRT basics to the neurodivergent brain in menopause. Grounded in current evidence and updated regularly.

A4M Blog—Anti-Aging Medicine Forum

blog.a4m.com

• Current clinical updates from A4M practitioners on hormone optimization, metabolic health, peptide therapy, and longevity medicine. Relevant to women tracking emerging options beyond standard hormone therapy, including developments in personalized lab testing and precision diagnostics.

IFM Blog—Institute for Functional Medicine

ifm.org/news-insights

- Practitioner-level articles on root-cause approaches to hormonal dysfunction, gut-hormone connections, thyroid health, adrenal support, and more. The IFM article on menopause hormone therapy weighing benefits and risks is an excellent complement to the NAMS position statements—it contextualizes the evidence within the whole-woman framework.

A Final Note on Information Quality

Menopause medicine is evolving quickly. What was standard guidance ten years ago is being revised, refined, and in some cases corrected—including, as you now know, the blanket warnings from the Women's Health Initiative that shaped an entire generation of clinical practice. This means that where you get your information matters enormously.

The resources above share a few things in common: they are grounded in peer-reviewed evidence, they are written or curated by clinicians with genuine specialization in this field, and they are regularly updated as the science develops. They will not all agree on every detail—medicine rarely does—but they will give you the tools to ask better questions, understand the answers, and advocate for yourself from a position of genuine knowledge.

That, in the end, is what all of this is for.

- Amber Bocknek, MD CCFP ABAARM FAAMM MSCP

Made in United States
Cleveland, OH
02 May 2026

36520585R00089